# Medical Transnationalism

# Korean Communities across the World

## **Series Editor:** Joong-Hwan Oh, Hunter College, CUNY

*Korean Communities across the World* publishes works that address aspects of (a) the Korean American community, (b) Korean society, (c) the Korean communities in other foreign lands, and (d) transnational Korean communities. In the field of (a) the Korean American community, this series welcomes contributions involving concepts such as Americanization, pluralism, social mobility, migration/immigration, social networks, social institutions, social capital, racism/discrimination, settlement, identity, and politics, as well as a specific topic related to family/marriage, gender roles, generations, work, education, culture, citizenship, health, ethnic community, housing, ethnic identity, racial relations, social justice, social policy, and political views, among others. In the field of (b) Korean society, this series embraces scholarship on current issues such as gender roles, age/aging, low fertility, immigration, urbanization, gentrification, economic inequality, high youth unemployment, sexuality, democracy, political power, social injustice, the nation's educational problems, social welfare, capitalism, consumerism, labor, health, housing, crime, environmental degradation, and the social life in the digital age and its impacts, among others. Contributors in the field of (c) Korean communities in other foreign lands are encouraged to submit works that expand our understanding about the formation, vicissitudes, and major issues of an ethnic Korean community outside of South Korea and the United States, such as cultural or linguistic retention, ethnic identity, assimilation, settlement patterns, citizenship, economic activities, family relations, social mobility, and racism/discrimination. Lastly, contributions relating to (d) transnational Korean communities may touch upon transnational connectivity in family, economy/finance, politics, culture, technology, social institutions, and people.

### Recent Titles

*Transnational Communities in the Smartphone Age: The Korean Community in the Nation's Capital*, by Dae Young Kim

*Medical Transnationalism: Korean Immigrants' Medical Tourism to South Korea*, by Sou Hyun Jang

*Transnational Return Migration of 1.5 Generation Korean New Zealanders: A Quest for Home*, by Jane Yeonjae Lee

# Medical Transnationalism

## Korean Immigrants' Medical Tourism to South Korea

Sou Hyun Jang

LEXINGTON BOOKS
*Lanham • Boulder • New York • London*

Published by Lexington Books
An imprint of The Rowman & Littlefield Publishing Group, Inc.
4501 Forbes Boulevard, Suite 200, Lanham, Maryland 20706
www.rowman.com

Unit A, Whitacre Mews, 26-34 Stannary Street, London SE11 4AB



Portions of this text were previously published as: Sou Hyun Jang. "Here or There: Recent US Immigrants' Medical and Dental Tourism and Associated Factors." International Journal of Health Services. Jang, Sou Hyun. "Here or There: Recent US Immigrants' Medical and Dental Tourism and Associated Factors." International Journal of Health Services 48, no. 1 (2018): 148–165. (online published September 27, 2017); Jang, Sou Hyun. "Factors Associated with Korean Immigrants' Medical Tourism to the Homeland." American journal of health behavior 41, no. 4 (2017): 461–470; and reprinted from Jang, Sou Hyun. "First-generation Korean immigrants' barriers to healthcare and their coping strategies in the US." Social Science & Medicine 168 (2016): 93–100, with permission from Elsevier.



British Library Cataloguing in Publication Information Available

**Library of Congress Cataloging-in-Publication Data**

Names: Jang, Sou Hyun, author.
Title: Medical transnationalism : Korean immigrants' medical tourism to South Korea / Sou Hyun Jang.
Description: Lanham : Lexington Books, 2018. | Series: Korean communities across the world | Includes bibliographical references and index.
Identifiers: LCCN 2018011447 (print) | LCCN 2018013581 (ebook) | ISBN 9781498563338 (Electronic) | ISBN 9781498563321 (cloth : alk. paper)
Subjects: LCSH: Medical tourism—Korea (South) | Immigrants—Medical care—Korea (South) | Emigration and immigration—Health aspects—Korea (South)
Classification: LCC RA793.5 (ebook) | LCC RA793.5 .J36 2018 (print) | DDC 362.1086/912095195—dc23
LC record available at https://lccn.loc.gov/2018011447

∞™ The paper used in this publication meets the minimum requirements of American National Standard for Information Sciences—Permanence of Paper for Printed Library Materials, ANSI/NISO Z39.48-1992.

Printed in the United States of America

# Contents

# Acknowledgments

It would not have been possible for me to publish this book without the support and guidance of Professor Pyong Gap Min at Queens College and the Graduate Center of the City University of New York (CUNY). For years, he has served as my "academic father," teaching me how to become an independent scholar. Whenever I wanted to give up, his encouragement inspired me to keep moving forward.

I also express my gratitude to Professor Paul Attewell and Mary Clare Lennon, who have provided useful suggestions on this study. Professor Joong Hwan Oh at Hunter College also read the book manuscript and gave me helpful comments. I am grateful to my editor, Sarah Craig, and her assistant, Julia Torres, at Lexington Books, who have been very supportive and understanding.

This is my book, but it also belongs to the Korean immigrants who were willing to join my study without any monetary rewards. I was surprised and grateful that most of them were open to talking about the very personal subject of their struggles and experiences in getting medical care, either in the United States or in the home country. I hope my research will contribute some of their situations to overcome their barriers to healthcare in the United States.

It was not easy to collect and analyze over 500 Korean survey respondents and 120 in-depth interviewees for this study. I was able to do so because many people helped me. I gratefully acknowledge my friend and a fellow sociologist Sejung Lim who helped me collect the survey data at various ethnic and community events. I would like to acknowledge that Young Oak Kim, In Ja Kim, Moon Young Chung, Jong Moo Cho, Yeo Oak Yoon, Hyun Ja Choi, Mi Kyung Noh, and Ji Ho Song helped me to collect the survey data and to arrange in-depth interviews.

Many friends at the Graduate Center, Fang Xu, Anna Gjika, Bronwyn Dobchuk-land, Erin Michaels, Dominique Nisperos, David Monaghan, and Chunrye Kim gave me emotional support. Thomas Chung, my good friend, helped me editing the first version of this book. Professor Robin Isserles has been a great mentor to me and has offered advice not only about being a scholar but also about how to have a balanced life as both a scholar and a mother. My "social transnational ties" helped me in writing this book; I am grateful to my best friends in Korea, Kyung Eun Lee, Sun Hee Lee, and Yeon Ju Lee, who offered me tremendous emotional comfort and encouragement in this process.

I would especially like to acknowledge the support and love of my family. My parents, Hyo Eun Seo and Se Yang Jang, gave me unconditional love and unwavering support. I am very glad that I am able to dedicate this book to my parents. I appreciate my brother, Won Ik Jang who was always there for me when I needed someone to talk to. I also thank Myung Sook Chung and San Keun Oh, my parents-in-law, for their support and prayers for me.

The smiles of my two sons, Phillip and Henry, were my greatest strength in effort of writing and revising the manuscript. Finally, my deepest appreciation goes to my husband and soulmate, Hyung Il Oh. I know we will always remember and talk about the nights we spent quietly writing together at the dinner table while our two boys were sleeping.

# Introduction

## BACKGROUND

Globalization has brought many new social phenomena that have changed peoples' lives. One new phenomenon that has emerged is international medical tourism: trips abroad to obtain medical services. These trips are usually from more developed countries such as those in North America, Western Europe, and the Middle East to less developed countries such as Mexico, India, Thailand, Singapore, and South Korea (Korea) (Connell 2006; De Arellano 2007; Gahlinger 2008; Ko 2011; Reed 2008). Many scholars have pointed out that this worldwide phenomenon has grown rapidly in recent years (Balaban and Marano 2010; Connell 2006; Green 2008; Mattoo and Rathindran 2006). Focusing on the US context, Keckley and Underwood (2008) predicted that the number of American medical tourists would increase to about 16 million by 2017.

Before I begin this book, I need to clarify how I define medical tourism and participants who engage in medical tourism. Several scholars (Garcia-Altes 2005; Lunt and Carrera 2010) have distinguished medical tourism from health tourism; they claim that medical tourism is derived from health tourism, a broader term that encompasses improving, maintaining, and recovering individual well-being. Although there seems to be no commonly agreed definition of medical tourism, scholars commonly use two conditions to define it: (1) individuals travel from their country to another foreign country, and (2) this trip is intended to get medical care and services.

Foreign-born immigrants show a greater propensity for medical tourism than native-born Americans due to high medical costs in the United States, unfamiliarity with the US healthcare system, and lack of health insurance (Reed 2008; US Department of Commerce 2005; Wallace,

Mendez-Luck, and Castañeda 2009). Despite their greater tendency to take medical tours than the general population, there is no consensus on how to define immigrants' medical tourism. Their visit to the home country for medical care is also called *diaspora medical tourism* (Keckley and Underwood 2008; Reed 2008; Xing 1998) or *medical return* (Bergmark, Barr, and Garcia 2010; Horton and Cole 2011). However, in this book, the term *medical tourism* is used because it is the most suitable term to define the subject of my research in this book: immigrants' visit to their home country with the intention of medical care or treatment, but not solely for the medical purpose.

Some long-term visitors to foreign countries might visit a doctor's office or a hospital for medical care when they fall ill or become injured. For example, one interviewee visited an acupuncturist office several times during his stay in Seoul for one month because he had severe back pain caused by his holding two pieces of heavy luggage at the airport. However, these people cannot be considered true medical tourists. The OECD (2011) refers to them as *unfortunate tourists*, not *medical tourists*. Thus, I consider immigrants as *medical tourists* when they meet the following two conditions. First of all, they should have intended to get medical care prior to their visits to the home country. Second, the participants should have received major medical treatments in the home country, such as surgeries, physical examinations, and dental care.

Since this book examines Korean immigrants' medical tours to their home country, it is also important to know how the Korean government defines people who visit Korea specifically to obtain medical care. The Korean government calls them *foreign patients* (KHIDI 2010). There are three criteria to be considered a foreign patient by the Korean government's definition: (1) the individual should not have Korean citizenship, (2) the individual should not have Korean national health insurance, and (3) the individual should not be registered as a foreigner with the Korean government. Thus, Korean immigrants who maintain Korean citizenship with the US permanent residency are not considered foreign patients by the Korean government. However, this book encompasses all Korean residents in the United States who include temporary residents, permanent residents, and naturalized US citizens because all these three groups can visit Korea for medical treatment. In this book, I refer to Korean immigrants who have visited the home country for medical care as *medical tourists* rather than foreign patients because their home country is not the true foreign country to them. Moreover, they do not meet the criteria of being foreign patients by the definition of the Korean government. However, I refer to foreigners who have visited Korea for medical care as foreign patients in chapter 2 because that is how they are called by the Korean government and private sector agencies.

## THE NEED FOR THE STUDY

Despite the greater propensity for medical tourism among immigrants than the native-born and the plausible reasons for engaging in it, not many studies have systematically examined immigrants' medical tourism experiences. This is likely due to the recency of the medical tourism phenomenon in general and the difficulty of collecting data for one particular immigrant group. For example, popular health-related national data, such as the National Health Interview Survey (NHIS), do not reflect any questions about medical tourism. The New Immigrant Survey (NIS), provided by Princeton University, asks whether immigrants have seen a doctor in a foreign country, but the number of each ethnic group is not large enough for meaningful statistical analysis (e.g., the total number of Korean immigrants is less than 120).

Moreover, the vast majority of studies on immigrants' medical tourism has focused on Mexican immigrants due to the geographic proximity from the United States to Mexico and their low health insurance rates (Bergmark, Barr, and Garcia 2010; Brown 2008; Horton and Cole 2011; Landeck and Garza 2003). Only a few articles have covered other immigrant groups, including Chinese and Indian immigrants (Fong 2008; Lee, Kearns, and Friesen 2010; Xing 1998). Little effort has been made to examine general immigrants' or one particular immigrant group's medical tourism experience in one book.

Korea has become one of the world's "hot destinations for medical tourism" (CNN 2009; Horowitz, Rosensweig, and Jones 2007; Ko 2011), but Korea has not yet received as much attention as other strong medical tourism countries, such as India, Thailand, and Singapore (Choe 2008). Among the source countries of medical tourists to Korea, Americans make up one of the largest medical tourist groups. The 2010 report published by the Korea Health Industry Development Institute (KHIDI) showed that about 82,000 medical tourists visited Korea and that US medical tourists accounted for 32% of them. However, I assume that the number of US medical tourists might be undercounted because this Korean government report did not include Koreans who have US permanent residency or who are temporary residents of the United States. Another government report (KOTRA 2009) indicated that the Korean government and medical tourism agencies have targeted Korean immigrants rather than Caucasians in the United States, although the statistics on Korean immigrant medical tourists has not been collected by the Korean government.

Although the Korean media has paid attention to Korean immigrants' medical tourism to the home country, previous studies in academia include Korean immigrants in only a few English-speaking countries: New Zealand, Canada, and the United States. Lee, Kearns, and Friesen (2010) examined the medical tourism of Korean immigrants in New Zealand. However, the number of foreign patients from New Zealand is negligible. Wang and Kwak (2015) studied the medical tourism experience of Korean immigrants in Canada, but Canadian patients make up only a very small proportion of total foreign patients to Korea (KHIDI 2013). Finally, several scholars (Ko et al. 2016; Oh et al. 2014) examined the medical tourism of Korean immigrants in the United States, but these studies are restricted to the middle-aged and elderly Korean immigrants with particular types of medical services in the home country. Thus, this book will contribute to the scarce literature on Korean immigrant medical tourists to Korea, as it encompasses all ages and genders and analyzes a large-scale survey and in-depth personal interviews.

## MAIN OBJECTIVES

This book intends to bridge the gap in research on Korean immigrants' medical tourism to the home country using relevant sociological theories and research methods. It has three main interrelated objectives. First, it examines how the Korean government's policy and its close coordination with private sector agencies have contributed to the development of medical tourism to Korea since the mid-2000s. It also examines the extent to which government agencies and medical organizations in Korea have targeted Korean immigrants in the United States and foreign patients from other countries.

Second, this book answers the following questions regarding Korean immigrants' barriers to formal US healthcare and their healthcare behaviors in the United States: What are the barriers for Korean immigrants to receive medical care in the United States? Do these barriers contribute to their distinct healthcare behaviors? How are these barriers and behaviors associated with their decision regarding medical tours to the home country? Third, what are the other contributing factors to their medical tourism? To answer these questions, I first probe into their barriers to the US healthcare and their healthcare behaviors in the United States, which are closely related to their decision regarding medical tourism to Korea. Then I examine whether Korean immigrants' transnational ties with the home country, their health insurance status, temporary resident status, socioeconomic status, and other demographic characteristics affect their decisions on medical tourism.

Lastly, this book explores several aspects of Korean immigrant medical tourists' experiences during their medical tourism and their evaluation of medical tourism after they have experienced it. It investigates the arrangements and processes of their medical tourism, the places where they received medical services, and the types of medical care obtained in Korea. It also investigates the level of their satisfaction with medical care in Korea compared to medical costs and medical services obtained in the

United States, as well as their future plans to revisit the home country for medical care.

## THEORETICAL AND CONCEPTUAL FRAMEWORKS

### Transnationalism Theory

Used by immigration scholars, transnationalism or transnational ties refer to the extent to which immigrants or immigrant organizations maintain linkages to their home countries. Some scholars have not made a clear distinction between transnationalism in general and immigrant transnationalism in particular. For example, Portes and his colleagues' 1999 article placed general transnationalism as its analytic center whereas his 2001 study gave answers to many questions related to immigrants' transnationalism in particular. In this book, I focus on immigrants' transnationalism rather than transnationalism in general.

Social science research on contemporary immigrants' transnational ties began in the early 1990s (Basch, Schiller, and Blanc 1994; Schiller, Basch, and Blanc Szanton 1992). In 1994, Basch and her colleagues defined transnationalism "as the processes by which immigrants forge and sustain multi-stranded relations that link together their societies of origin and settlement" (Basch, Schiller, and Blanc 1994, 7). Following their pioneering work, many sociologists and other social scientists have conducted research on immigrant transnational ties (Foner 1997; Itzigsohn 2000; Kasinitz et al. 2002; Levitt 2001; Levitt and Waters 2002; Levitt, DeWind, and Vertovec 2003; Min 2012b; Portes 2003; Portes, Guarnizo, and Landolt 1999; Smith 2005; Smith and Guarnizo 1998).

Portes and his colleagues have applied a narrow definition of transnational ties that includes only "occupations and activities that require regular and sustained social context over time across borders for their implementations" (Portes, Guarnizo, and Landolt 1999, 219). However, other scholars have used a broader definition, including immigrants' economic, political, social, and cultural activities with their homelands (Faist 2000; Itzigsohn et al. 1999; Itzigsohn 2000). Korean immigrants' medical tourism to the home country does not belong to the narrow definition of medical transnationalism because it does not require regular visits to the home country. Their medical tours to the home country might be a onetime trial. However, it can be still considered as a form of transnationalism because it requires their actual visits to Korea.

Broadly used, transnationalism indicates individual, organizational, or governmental cross-border activities. Scholars have distinguished transnationalism with the high and low levels of institutionalization (Schiller,

Basch, and Blanc Szanton 1992; Guarnizo and Smith 1998; Portes 2001). According to them, *transnationalism from below* refers to everyday transnational practices or bottom-up grassroots movements at the individual level, whereas *transnationalism from above* means top-down transnational activities at government or corporate level. However, this binary categorization of transnationalism has been criticized by several researchers (Chin and Smith 2015; Waldinger and Fitzgerald 2004) because the notion of *transnationalism from above* regards nation-states as passive and powerless. Instead, Chin and Smith (2015) argued that nation-states are essential and active entities that can initiate, promote, and maintain transnational activities. They pointed out that *state transnationalism*, transnational activities that were launched or supported by states, happens when the state seeks its national interests. They also indicated that state transnationalism does not need to be top-down; it includes cooperation between the homeland states and diaspora communities. The Korean government's and other private sectors' efforts to attract Korean immigrants to the home country for medical care can be considered as state transnationalism because it is initiated and actively promoted by the Korean government in its pursuit of national economic interests. The concept of state transnationalism is applied in chapter 2 when I explore the Korean government's strategies to attract foreign patients, including Korean immigrants.

Previously, Portes and other transnational scholars have classified immigrants' transnational activities into the following forms: economic, political, social, and cultural (Itzigsohn 2000; Kivisto 2003; Portes 2001). As another form of transnational activities, some immigration scholars have studied US immigrants' transnational religious activities, which involve connecting their host cities of settlement and their home cities, both individually or organizationally (Levitt 2001; McAlister 1998; Min 2010). In contrast to the plethora of research on these types of immigrant transnationalism, there have been only a few studies of immigrants' medical transnational ties with the home country. For example, Portes, Fernández-Kelly, and Light (2012, 16) considered medical transnationalism as one of the coping strategies when legal immigrants have temporary difficulties in getting health insurance for formal healthcare in the United States. They gave an example of Latino immigrants' crossing borders for a temporary return to their home country with the intention of receiving medical care. Although they indicated immigrants' medical tourism to their home countries as an example of medical transnationalism, they have not explored it with any empirical data.

Considering immigrants only, there are narrow and broad definitions of medical transnationalism. On the one hand, a narrow definition of medical transnationalism includes immigrants visiting the home country to get medical care. This form adheres to the narrow definition of medical transnationalism because it requires the physical movement of an individual immigrant to the home country with the intention of getting medical care. Unlike the broad definition of medical transnationalism, which will be explained later, this narrow type is deeply connected with other types of transnationalism. For example, it is associated with dual citizenship among immigrants, which is a form of political transnationalism. Immigrants who have dual citizenship of both their home and receiving countries might visit their home country more often and more easily. Thus, their chance of getting medical care in the home country might increase as well. Social and cultural transnationalism are also related to immigrants' medical tourism. Relatives or friends in the home country can help making medical appointments for immigrants even before they arrive the home country so that they can get medical care more quickly and easily. Moreover, seeing advertisements on ethnic media such as television, newspapers, and radio in the receiving countries can make immigrants more likely to consider a medical tour to their home country. The associations between Korean immigrants' medical tourism with different types of transnationalism will be examined in detail in chapter 4.

On the other hand, a broad definition of medical transnationalism includes all other types that do not require immigrants' actual visit to the home country. Receiving medicine from the home country or consulting health information from the home country can be considered as examples of the broad definition of immigrant medical transnationalism. Since a broad medical transnationalism has weak ties with other types of transnationalism, this book does not cover this broad type.

## Theories and Concepts on Immigrants' Healthcare Utilization

Since medical tourism can be considered as one of the healthcare utilization options, several theories and concepts related to immigrants' healthcare utilization are applied to examine their medical tourism in this book. Andersen (1968, 1973, and 1995) provided one of the most popular healthcare utilization models for the general population. He (1968, 1995) and his colleague Newman (1973) suggested that there are three factors that determine healthcare services: (1) predisposing factors (e.g., sociodemographic characteristics such as race, gender, and age), (2) enabling factors (e.g., access to healthcare and ability to pay for healthcare such as having health insurance, social relationships involving support from family and community), and (3) perceived and actual need for health service.

Although Andersen's model is one of the widely known models in healthcare utilization for the general population, there is a limitation to this model because it was not specifically designed for immigrants. Nevertheless, applying Andersen's framework, Akresh (2009) found that this model was not exclusive to examination of the general population's healthcare utilization; it also applied to examination of immigrants' healthcare utilization with several immigrant factors. When Andersen's framework was used, various factors were associated with Latino and Asian immigrants' healthcare utilization and dental care utilization in the United States. For example, several enabling factors (e.g., years living in the United States and health insurance status) have been commonly and positively associated with both groups' healthcare utilization. However, a level of English proficiency has been associated only with Asian immigrants' healthcare utilization. Immigrants' medical tourism might have different features from a typical healthcare behavior in the United States because the foreign countries have different healthcare systems and culture than the United States. Nonetheless, it will be interesting to see whether Andersen's framework applies to immigrants' medical tourism, which typically has not been recognized as a normal healthcare utilization behavior, but can still be considered a type of healthcare utilization behavior.

Some researchers argued that there are barrier factors more relevant to immigrants who are more vulnerable and more likely to show underutilization or delayed utilization than the general population (Carrasquillo, Carrasquillo, and Shea 2000; Derose, Escarce, and Lurie 2007; Derose et al. 2009; Ell and Castaneda 1998; Leclere, Jensen, and Biddlecom 1994). They have pointed out that immigrants' barriers to healthcare can be categorized into three: (1) structural, (2) financial, and (3) personal barriers. In chapter 1, I thoroughly review what kinds of barriers Korean immigrants face in the United States, while I review barriers that apply to immigrants in general here.

First, structural barriers include limited chances to meet doctors who share the same culture, language, and race/ethnic background. An individual is more likely to choose a doctor of the individual's same race or ethnicity (Gray and Stoddard 1997; LaVeist and Nuru-Jeter 2002; Saha et al. 1999), and to feel higher satisfaction with the doctor-patient relationship if the doctor and patient share the same culture and language (LaVeist and Nuru-Jeter 2002; Saha et al. 1999). However, immigrants tend to be less likely to interact with doctors who share the same race, ethnic language, and culture due to the small number of minority physicians. For example, white Americans show a much higher percentage of patient-physician racial concordance (86%) than African-Americans (22%), Hispanic Americans (19%), and Asian-Americans (52%) (LaVeist and Nuru-Jeter 2002; LaVeist, Nuru-Jeter, and Jones 2003). This circumstance may lead to misunderstanding and frustration for minority and immigrant patients (Kraut 1990; LaVeist and Nuru-Jeter 2002; LaVeist, Nuru-Jeter, and Jones; Takada et al. 1998). Structural barriers also include geographic proximity to hospitals, locations of hospitals, and access to public or private transportation to hospitals.

Second, there are financial barriers to immigrants' healthcare that include poverty, lack of financial resources, or lack of health insurance. Many scholars found that immigrants' uninsured status plays a negative role in their healthcare access (Derose, Escarce, and Lurie 2007; Derose et al. 2009; Jang, Kim, and Chiriboga 2005). Lastly, personal barriers such as the level of acculturation (Arcia et al. 2001; Gorman, Read, and Krueger 2010; Salant and Lauderdale 2003), perceived discrimination (Jang, Kim, and Chiriboga 2005; Viruell-Fuentes 2007; Yoo, Gee, and Takeuchi 2009), limited language proficiency (Hu and Covell, 1986; Jang, Kim, and Chiriboga; Kim et al. 2011; Wu, Kviz, and Miller 2009), and cultural differences (Jenkins et al. 1996; Kung, 2004; Wu, Kviz, and Miller 2009) have been associated with lack of access to healthcare. In particular, previous studies found that culture and language have a big impact on the provision of healthcare, such as the doctor-patient relationship (Ferguson and Candib 2002; Flores 2000; LaVeist and Nuru-Jeter 2002) and the use of complementary and alternative medicine (CAM) (Bodeker and Kronenberg 2002; Hsiao et al. 2006; Kronenberg et al. 2006; Ma 1999), especially among minority patients.

Some previous studies pointed out that immigrants' barriers to access to formal healthcare utilization contributed to their coping strategies, such as going to free clinics, seeing co-ethnic doctors (Choi 2013; Portes, Fernández-Kelly, and Light 2012; Wang 2007; Wang, Rosenberg, and Lo 2008), usage of folk medicine (Akresh 2009; Han 2001; Hill et al. 2006; Kim and Chan 2004; Portes, Fernández-Kelly, and Light 2012; Pourat et al. 1999; Wu, Burke, and LeBaron 2007), or medical tours to the home country (Brown 2008; Landeck and Garza 2003; Lee, Kearns, and Friesen 2010; Oh et al. 2014; Wang and Kwak 2015). Notably, Portes, Fernández-Kelly, and Light (2012) set the framework for immigrants' different coping strategies based on their different types of barriers to access to formal US healthcare. According to their categorization, there are four possible situations based on the types of barriers and coping strategies. First, when immigrants lack English proficiency or have cultural differences, they tend to see co-ethnic healthcare professionals as a coping strategy. Second, when immigrants are uninsured, they tend to seek folk medicine or see unlicensed doctors. Third, if recent immigrants are not able to access federal health programs, such as Medicaid or Medicare, they tend to go back to the home country for medical care or use free clinics. Lastly, undocumented immigrants tend to seek folk healers, go to free clinics, or receive drugs from the home country. Applying Portes and his associates' frameworks, chapter 3 will examine if and how these barriers contribute to Korean immigrants' medical tour to the home country as one of their coping strategies.

## DATA SOURCES AND RESEARCH METHODS

Use of multiple data sources is a major strength of this book. I used the following data sources: (1) public documents, (2) my own survey of 507 Korean immigrants, (3) personal interviews with 20 staff members representing various groups in New York and Korea, (4) audio-taped personal interviews with 100 Korean immigrant participants in medical tourism to Korea and 20 nonparticipants, and (5) Korean- and local English-language newspaper articles. The first two data sources offered quantitative data while the last three offered qualitative data.

### Public Documents

I used the 2009–2011 American Community Surveys (ACS) to analyze Korean immigrants' demographic (e.g., gender, age, and citizenship status) and socioeconomic characteristics (e.g., educational level and occupational characteristics), and the rate of health insurance. I combined the 2009–2011 ACS data from the Integrated Public Use Microdata Series (IPUMS). I chose this data period because the Census Bureau began to include the health insurance variables in 2008. When I analyzed the data, I mainly compared three groups: foreign-born Koreans with native-born Koreans and native-born non-Hispanic whites. The Korean sample includes only single-race Korean respondents.

### Survey of Korean Immigrants in the NY-NJ Area

This book analyzed the survey data of 507 Korean immigrants. The participants include first-generation Korean immigrant adults who are 18 years and older and who came to the United States at age 13 or older. The survey participants were recruited in the New York-New Jersey (NY-NJ) metropolitan area, which has the second largest concentration of Korean immigrants in the United States. They were recruited from ethnic-religious organizations, major ethnic festivals (e.g., Korean Parade in Manhattan, Korean Thanksgiving, Folklore Festival in Queens, and Korean Festival in New Jersey), other ethnic events at the ethnic community centers, and personal channels between fall 2013 and spring 2014. Non-probability sampling techniques were applied in this book because it was not feasible to secure a list of all Korean immigrants in the NY-NJ area. Instead, a quota sampling technique was used to select survey participants by gender, educational level, class of work, age, and religious background to match the demographic, socioeconomic, and religious characteristics of Korean immigrants.

The survey questionnaire included about 40 items. The items can be classified in the following categories: (1) demographic and socioeconomic characteristics and immigration history, (2) involvement in Korean networks and associations, (3) health insurance and other health-related issues, (4) transnational activity, and (5) medical tourism to Korea. The characteristics of survey respondents are provided in the Appendix. To measure Korean immigrants' medical tourism, I asked all of my survey respondents, "Have you ever visited Korea for medical care since you migrated to the United States?" I asked them to say no to this question if they received medical care accidentally without any plan prior to their trip. Then, I asked follow-up questions to those who said yes to the prior question, such as frequency of their medical tourism and the year of their last visit to the home country for medical care.

The survey was self-administered and paper-based. On average, respondents took about 20 minutes to complete the survey, and no monetary reward was offered to the respondents. All answers from the survey data were coded and analyzed by the author using Stata 13. A chi-squared test was conducted in (see Chapter 3 and 4) to examine the association between possible contributing factors and Korean immigrants' medical tours to the home country.

## Personal Interviews with Local Staff Members

I interviewed 20 staff members of various organizations in the Korean community in New York and in Korea: (1) Korean travel agencies in New York, (2) Korean community centers in New York, (3) Ministry of Health and Welfare, and (4) three hospitals (Seoul Asan, Yonsei Severance, and Inha University hospitals) in Korea that had received foreign patients and Korean immigrant medical tourists. I asked several questions to these staff members to get background information about when the medical tourism started, how prevalent it is, the proportion of overseas Koreans out of all foreign patients, how the participants are recruited, common types of medical services that the participants have received, how much money they spend and how they pay, the strategies of each agency to attract more medical tourists, and other related issues. The interview contents were analyzed in chapter 2 to examine the Korean government's and private sector agencies' efforts to attract foreign patients.

## Audio-taped Personal Interviews with 120 Korean Immigrant Participants

A small number of survey respondents was willing to respond to further open-ended questions immediately following the survey. However, the majority of survey participants refused to do so. Since it was hard to find a sufficient number of interviewees through the survey, a snowball sampling technique was used to recruit more informants. A small number of initial interviewees was recruited at Korean ethnic churches and Korean community centers in the NY-NJ area. In order to reduce the bias of having certain group of Korean immigrants as interviewees, I categorized Korean immigrants into five groups: (1) international students, (2) young Koreans who are between 18 and 29 years old, (3) adult Koreans who are between 30 and 44 years old, (4) middle-aged Koreans who are between 45 and 64 years old, and (5) elderly Koreans who are 65 years old or older. I tried to make almost equal numbers of interviewees for each group and balanced numbers of men and women in each group. I believe this categorization helped me to analyze and compare how sociodemographic characteristics (e.g., age, gender, occupation, and visa status) of each group contribute to their medical tourism experiences.

Eventually, I conducted audio-taped personal interviews with 100 Korean immigrants who had taken at least one medical tour to Korea. I also talked with 20 non-medial tourists and asked them why they had not engaged in medical tourism to Korea. I included those nonparticipants for comparison of their decision and experience of medical tourism to those of the participants. However, my in-depth interviews mostly focused on medical tourists who had been to Korea and received medical treatments or services at least once. I asked them about their medical tourism experiences in detail. Although I included questions about medical tourism in the survey questionnaire, personal interviews gave me more detailed and nuanced information about the experience of medical tourism than survey questions.

About 50 questions, mostly open-ended, were asked of the informants. These questions probed into the participants' background characteristics, including information about their health insurance, the factors that contributed to their decision to take medical tours, the duration of their medical tours, the types of healthcare received in Korea, their evaluations of the quality of medical services obtained in Korea for the cost, and their plan to continue to use medical tours for their medical care.

Each in-depth interview took about 30 minutes to an hour to complete. All audio-recorded interviews were conducted in Korean, translated into English, and transcribed in Word 2013 by the author. The qualitative data was analyzed manually instead of using a software program. Contents of in-depth interviews were categorized by assigning a number to important keywords (e.g., language barrier, health insurance, and co-ethnic doctor) then analyzed by the keyword and the interviewee's sociodemographic characteristics. Every name appearing in this book is a pseudonym. I believe that the audio-taped personal interviews are the central component of data for this book and provide many interesting comments from the informants.

### Korean- and English-Language Daily Newspaper Articles

Finally, I collected and analyzed newspaper articles published in the *Korea Daily* and *Korea Times,* the two Korean-language daily newspapers published in the NY-NJ area to gain perspectives of the Korean and Korean American communities. I also collected and reviewed articles from *Chosun Ilbo* and *Joongang Ilbo*, the two newspapers in Korea with the most subscribers. Scholars (Ko 2011; Reddy, York, and Brannon 2010) have noted the media has shown more interest in medical tourism than academia. Thus, newspaper articles can show how discourses on medical tourism have changed over time. Since the Korean government has begun to promote medical tourism since 2009, I expected to find different types of articles on medical tourism before and after that year. Thus, I collected articles published in four Korean-language daily newspapers published in Korea and the United States from January 1, 2003, to December 31, 2016, using the keyword *medical tourism* on each newspaper's archival website. Contents of newspaper articles were categorized by assigning a number to important keywords (e.g., foreign patients, cosmetic surgery), then analyzed by the keyword.

## STRUCTURE OF THE BOOK

This book consists of an introduction, five substantive chapters, and a conclusion. Introduction first briefly describes medical tourism as a recent global phenomenon and why its study is needed. It then provides the main objectives of this book and its theoretical frameworks. It also clarifies research methods and major data sources. Finally, Introduction summarizes the organization of this book.

Chapter 1 (Literature Review and Background Information) reviews the literature on medical tourism and provides background information on Korean immigrants in the United States. The first section of this chapter reviews previous studies of medical tourism in general, such as its various definitions and types. It then examines the previous studies of different immigrants' medical tourism to the home country. It also reviews Korean immigrants' various barriers to formal US healthcare and their various healthcare patterns in the United States, including their medical tourism to Korea. The second section of this chapter provides background information about Korean immigrants. Based on the existing literature and the ACS data, it covers Korean immigrants' socioeconomic characteristics, concentration in small businesses, ethnic attachment, health-related issues, and transnational ties with the home country.

Chapter 2 (The Development of Medical Tourism in Korea and the Related Issues) investigates the development of medical tourism in Korea and the

Korean government's effort to promote the medical tourism industry in Korea. This chapter pays particular attention to government agencies' and the private sector's efforts and strategies to attract more foreign patients and to bring more Korean immigrants to Korea for medical care. It also explores economic and social changes brought by medical tourism along with problems caused by medical tourism. In this chapter, I mainly use secondary resources, such as newspaper articles, reports by government agencies, and results of social science research on medical tourism.

Chapter 3 (Korean Immigrants' Healthcare Behaviors in the United States) examines Korean immigrants' barriers to formal US healthcare and their healthcare behaviors based on results of a major survey and in-depth personal interviews. I focus on three major healthcare behaviors: Korean immigrants' preference and dependence on co-ethnic doctors, their practice of *Hanbang* (traditional Korean medicine), and their medical tourism to the home country. I examine why Korean immigrants show these healthcare behaviors and how the first two behaviors are related to the last one: medical tourism.

Chapter 4 (Factors Contributing to Korean Immigrants' Medical Tourism) shows the prevalence of Korean immigrants' medical tourism. It then attempts to explain the factors contributing to Korean immigrants' decisions on medical tourism, paying special attention to medical tourism participants' transnational characteristics, health insurance status, legal status, and other characteristics. As major data sources, I use in-depth personal interviews with participants in addition to the survey data.

Chapter 5 (Korean Immigrants' Medical Tourism Experience and Evaluation) focuses on medical tourism participants' experiences during their stay in the home country for medical care and their evaluation of it. It provides information about the arrangement of Korean immigrants' medical tourism, the duration of their medical tourism, the types of medical care they receive in Korea, and the cities chosen for medical treatments. It also examines Korean medical tourists' evaluations of medical tourism and future plans to revisit Korea for medical care. Along with chapters 3 and 4, this chapter will be the most important chapter in this book because it will contribute new findings on Korean immigrants' medical tourism based on my own data.

Conclusion summarizes the major findings, discusses their theoretical and practical contributions, and suggests a typology of Korean immigrant medical tourists based on the two important contributing factors. It also recommends policy implications for the Korean Community in the United States and the US government.

# *Chapter 1*

# Literature Review and Background Information

## A REVIEW OF LITERATURE ON MEDICAL TOURISM

### Medical Tourism in General

Medical tourism is not an entirely new phenomenon; people have traveled in search of better, cheaper, or more comfortable healthcare. However, it is a new term in the globalization era and had not received much attention until recently. Moreover, academic researchers have shown much less interest in medical tourism than the public and private sectors have shown (Ko 2011; Reddy, York, and Brannon 2010). In addition to the relative scarcity of academic research, scholars have pointed out that the inconsistent definitions, lack of theoretical frameworks, and limited data pose difficulties in studying medical tourism (Balaban and Marano 2010; Lunt and Carrera 2010, Ko 2011; Reddy, York, and Brannon 2010; Reed 2008).

There seem to be no official US national data or national report that captures the exact number of medical tourists or their characteristics, although some studies have discussed the frequency of medical tourism or the characteristics of medical tourists based on their own survey data. For instance, in their 2008 report, Keckley and Underwood indicated that only 3% of their American survey participants had actually visited a foreign country to get medical treatment, but about 27% of the respondents indicated that they might do so in the future. Regarding the characteristics of outbound US patients, Asians are more likely to visit a foreign country to get elective care (i.e., procedures not directly related to a medical emergency), whereas the elderly and those with Medicare and Medicaid are less likely to do so. Horowitz, Rosensweig, and Jones (2007) explained that middle-class Americans without health insurance are the most likely to be medical tourists to a foreign country. By analyzing a survey data, Fisher and Sood (2014) found that about 15% of their survey respondents had taken medical tours to a foreign country, and the medical cost was the most influential factor in their medical tourism. According to their analysis, individuals who are younger, employed, and have had international travel experience are more likely to be engaged in medical tourism than their counterparts.

Most recent medical tourism studies seem to lean more toward a business perspective rather than a sociological perspective. For example, rather than exploring social issues caused by medical tourism, recent studies have examined the benefits to medical tourists of staying at a medical hotel (Han and Hyun 2014); compared the websites of hospitals attracting foreign patients (Moghavvemi et al. 2017); built a model to explain medical tourists' retention, which is influenced by quality, satisfaction, and trust (Han and Hyun 2015); developed a medical tourism index (Fetscherin and Stephano 2016); and analyzed the problems of medical tourism broker websites (Lee et al. 2013). Most of these studies have been published in tourism, marketing, or management journals, rather than social science journals.

Furthermore, the most recent academic publications include studies examining medical tourism in a particular country or receiving countries' strategies to attract more medical tourists. Since several Asian countries are currently among the most likely destinations of individuals who want to receive medical care in foreign countries, they have focused on the efforts and strategies of those countries, such as Singapore, India, Thailand, and Malaysia (Ganguli and Ebrahim 2017; Lee and Park 2013; Moghavvemi et al. 2017; Noree, Hanefeld, and Smith 2016; Ormond, Mun, and Khoon 2014; Sultana et al. 2014; Tang and Lau 2017; Wong, Velasamy, and Arshad 2014). Some Asian countries' strategies to promote medical tourism will be extensively reviewed in chapter 2, where I examine the development of medical tourism in Korea and the Korean government's efforts.

Scholars have pointed out that in addition to its benefits, such as cheaper medical expenses or the opportunity for sightseeing in foreign nations, medical tourism also may cause several potential risks and problems. First, it can be difficult for medical tourists to find good doctors and hospitals in a foreign country due to their limited knowledge and resources (Horowitz, Rosensweig, and Jones 2007). Second, it could be problematic for medical tourists to receive follow-up treatment or continuous medical care after a medical tour to a foreign country (Horowitz, Rosensweig, and Jones 2007; MacReady 2007). For example, if there is a side effect of medical care received in a foreign country, it would be difficult for medical tourists to return to the country where they received the treatment due to the cost and time involved. The limitation associated with follow-up treatment is a more serious issue especially among those who receive surgeries, such as transplant surgeries, in foreign countries (Canales, Kasiske, and Rosenberg 2006; Terzi, Kern, and Kohnen 2008). Moreover, as the doctors in a home country may feel not responsible for follow-up treatment after a surgery, the medical tourists may get lost between the two countries (Boschert 2007).

## US Immigrants' Medical Tourism to the Home Country

More researchers have paid attention to Mexican immigrants' medical tourism than to that of any other immigrant group for the following reasons. First, Mexican immigrants make up a large proportion of immigrant medical tourists to their home country simply because they account for more than 20% of the total number of immigrants in the United States (Bergmark, Barr, and Garcia 2010; Horton and Cole 2011; Macias and Morales 2001). Second, due to their unstable job status and the high rate of employment in the informal underground economy, they have the lowest rate of health insurance among all immigrant groups (Bastida, Brown III, and Pagán 2008; Bergmark, Barr, and Garcia 2010; Brown 2008). Third, since Mexico is one of the closest countries to the United States, Mexican immigrants can easily visit their homeland for medical care.

Horton and Cole (2011) pointed out that Mexican immigrants' medical tours to the home country are not limited to those who live close to the Mexico border. Nonetheless, researchers have focused on the medical tour experiences of Mexican immigrants who reside in the border states. In other words, due to the physical proximity to Mexico of certain US states, such as California, Arizona, New Mexico, and Texas, researchers have shown more interest in medical tours among Mexican immigrants in these border states. In fact, using the 2001 California Health Interview Survey (CHIS) data, Wallace, Mendez-Luck, and Castañeda (2009) found that Mexican immigrants' chance of taking a medical tour increases the closer they live to the border. Earlier, Chavez et al. (1985) found that about 30% of Mexican immigrants residing in San Diego had visited Mexico for healthcare since their migration to the United States. Other studies have commonly indicated that about 14% of Mexican immigrants in the border states have visited Mexico for medical purposes. For example, Macias and Morales (2001) conducted a survey of Mexican immigrants who attended a health fair in the city of Lennox in South Los Angeles (LA) County. They found that 14% of respondents had crossed the border to Mexico for medical care during the past year. Homedes and LaBrec's (1991) study shows similar results; 14% of 400 Mexican women at the Arizona-Sonora border used Mexico as their regular source of healthcare. Thompson (1993) also found that 14% of 618 Mexican Americans in the Lower Rio Grande Valley in Texas had visited Mexico for the medical treatment.

Researchers have found several contributing factors to Mexican immigrants' high propensity of medical tourism. First, a key factor is the fact that medical costs are relatively cheaper in Mexico than in the United States (Brown 2008; Horton and Cole 2011; Landeck and Garza 2003; Macias and Morales 2001; Thompson 1993; Wallace, Mendez-Luck, and Castañeda 2009). Thompson (1993) found that 83% of Mexican immigrant respondents in Texas identified lower cost as the single most important contributing factor to their healthcare use in Mexico. Most studies of Mexican immigrants' medical tourism have found that cultural preference, language, and family custom are all considered relatively less important by these immigrants compared to the cheaper medical costs in Mexico. About 70% of Mexican immigrant respondents in California also indicated the low cost of medical care in Mexico as the most important reason for their decision to take a medical tour to their home country (Macias and Morales 2001).

In addition to the lower medical costs, Mexican immigrants' uninsured status in the United States (Brown 2008; Landeck and Garza 2003) and their familiarity with home-country medical treatments (Wallace, Mendez-Luck, and Castañeda 2009) are other important contributing factors to their decisions to engage in medical tourism. Horton and Cole (2011) emphasized several features that attracted their Mexican immigrant interviewees to visit the home country for medical care, including the speed of medical services and the better personal relationships between doctors and patients.

I presume that there are some common motivational factors that contribute to both Mexican and Korean immigrants' medical trips to their home country: lower healthcare costs, convenience and familiarity with the homeland medical care, and the lack of US health insurance. There are also differences in medical tourism between the two immigrant groups. For example, it takes more time and requires more money for Koreans than for Mexicans to go back to the homeland due to Korea's distance from the United States. Also, Korean immigrants generally have a much higher level of socioeconomic status than Mexican immigrants. Therefore, I considered these similarities and differences when analyzing my survey data and in-depth personal interviews.

Studies of other immigrant groups' medical tourism are scarce compared to those of Mexican immigrants' medical tourism. Messias's (2002) study examined medical transnationalism with the narratives of Brazilian immigrant women in the United States. She found that her Brazilian immigrant women respondents, mostly domestic or temporary workers, faced economic and cultural barriers to access to formal healthcare in the United States. Thus, they utilized informal healthcare in the United States or used transnational health resources, such as getting medication from Brazil, relying on other Brazilian health resources, or returning to the home country for medical care.

Only a few studies have examined Asian immigrants' medical tourism. For example, Bookman and Bookman (2007) indicated that the development of medical tourism in India had begun to attract participants from Indian diasporic communities. When overseas Indians visit their friends and family in India, they also receive medical care or health checkups because of India's lower medical costs and their cultural affinity for the Indian styles of medical care. Fong (2008) examined the unexpected medical return among Chinese sojourners in Ireland and the United Kingdom. However, although this qualitative study showed the experiences of three Chinese sojourners' medical returns to their home country, its interviewees were individuals who had no children, moved frequently, and had lived in the host country for only a limited period of time. Thus, these temporary residents have different characteristics from most other immigrants. Moreover, since none of the Chinese sojourners in this study returned to the receiving country after getting medical care in the home country, their behaviors cannot be considered to be true medical tourism. Emphasizing the effect of cultural affinity on medical tourism, Xing (1998) reported that overseas Chinese visited the home country for medical care because they believed in traditional Chinese medicine. Most of these overseas Chinese in Xing's study are from countries near China, such as Hong Kong, Macau, and Taiwan. Since there are only a few studies on other Asian immigrant groups' medical tourism to their homeland, this book will contribute to the existing literature on Asian immigrants' medical tour experiences.

## Korean Immigrants' Medical Tourism to the Home Country

As indicated earlier, the number of social science studies on Korean immigrants' medical tourism is limited. There are few government-published articles on Korean immigrants' medical tourism. In 2006, the Korean Ministry of Health and Welfare published a report based on its survey of 271 Korean Americans living in Pennsylvania, New Jersey, California, Texas, Virginia, and Georgia. This report showed that about 83% of Korean immigrants would go to Korea for cosmetic surgery and that 60% would consider going to Korea for dental care, back surgery, or infertility treatment if the cost were appropriate. The report also indicated that, due to cheaper medical costs in Korea, it is still cheaper for Korean Americans to get healthcare in Korea even when their round-trip flight and living expenses during their stay are considered.

Some studies have treated medical tourism as one of the healthcare utilization options among Korean immigrants (De Gagne et al. 2014; Son 2013). Son (2013) explained that the development of technologies and globalization has led Korean immigrant women to consider their home country as an option of alternative medical care. The majority of Korean immigrant women feel favorably toward a medical tour to Korea because of the cheaper, faster, and more comfortable medical care as well as cultural familiarity. Moreover, De Gagne et al. (2014) found that some middle-aged Korean immigrants do not buy health insurance because they have an alternative place to obtain medical care: the home country. In fact, a significant proportion of uninsured middle-aged Korean immigrants (23%) did not have health insurance because of the availability of medical tourism.

Most of the major studies on Korean immigrants engaging in medical tourism have been conducted in three English-speaking countries—New Zealand, Canada, and the United States. Several significant examples of such studies are listed below. First, Lee et al. (2010) conducted a study of the use of homeland medical services among Korean immigrants in New Zealand. Through interviews with six first-generation middle-aged Korean immigrants in New Zealand who had surgery in Korea, they found that Korean immigrants go back to Korea not only for "effective" reasons (e.g., better-quality doctors, high-brand hospitals with good equipment, and faster medical services) but also for "affective" reasons (e.g., thinking of the homeland as an emotional and therapeutic place). Korean immigrants' higher expectations of medical care services, the lack of cultural and language barriers, the lack of perceived racism, and their subjective feelings of being more accepted in their home country are the main reasons for their decisions to go back to Korea for medical care. Although the authors give plausible explanations for Korean immigrants' medical tourism from New Zealand to Korea, the interviewees comprised only middle-aged (40–55 years old) individuals who had received medical surgery in Korea. Thus, their study could not compare how the patient's age or the type of medical care received is associated with Korean immigrants' medical tourism.

Second, with transnationalism as their theoretical framework, Wang and Kwak (2015) investigated the barriers to Canadian healthcare and transnational healthcare utilization among Korean immigrants in Toronto. As detailed in Introduction, I argue that there are different types of medical transnationalism among immigrants, such as getting pharmaceuticals from the home country and visiting the home country to get medical care. Congruent with my classification, Wang and Kwak (2015) also suggested several types of transnational healthcare, including importing medications from Korea, consulting health information from Korea, and visiting Korea for actual medical care. According to this study, Korean immigrants in Canada face several barriers when they try to get formal Canadian healthcare. First, the long distance that must be traveled to see a Korean doctor can be a problem. Although Korean immigrants prefer to see Korean doctors who share their language and culture, the geographic barrier makes them difficult to reach. Second, insurance coverage is another reason for them to choose to travel to the home country for alternative medical care. It is true that the Canadian government offers public health insurance, but its coverage is limited and does not cover some types of medical care, such as eye care, dental care, and MRIs. Thus, many Korean immigrants take medical tours to Korea, which has relatively lower costs for these types of medical care. Lastly, Korean immigrants have sociocultural barriers to access to formal healthcare in Canada. As a minority, they have limited social networks and social support from family and the ethnic community. In particular, it is more difficult for those with children to see a doctor in Canada due to the need for childcare while they receive medical care. These barriers contribute to their medical tourism to Korea, despite its disadvantages, such as the associated travel costs and the difficulty of getting aftercare.

In the US context, Oh et al. (2014) conducted a semi-structured focus group with 34 first-generation Korean female immigrants over the age of 40 in the Washington, DC, metropolitan area. They found that cost-effectiveness was the most important factor contributing to Korean female immigrants' medical tours, especially for cancer screening. Better, faster, and more accessible medical services in Korea are other strong contributing factors. Moreover, their barriers to US medical care and other personal reasons, such as visiting family and friends in the home country or having more personal time, also influence their decisions to take medical tours. Korean ethnic media's active marketing is another push factor in Korean immigrants' choice to take medical tours to the home country. The authors pointed out that Korean immigrants were not fully aware of the possible negative aspects of medical tourism, such as the difficulties associated with timely care and follow-up treatments. More recently, Jun and Oh (2015) analyzed two Korean American newspapers as primary sources of information among Korean immigrants in the United States and found that articles positively frame medical tourism for their readers.

The latest study of Korean Americans in the greater Seattle area (Ko et al. 2016) examined the association between colorectal cancer (CRC) screening and medical tourism, as well as contributing factors to Korean Americans' medical tours to the home country. Analyzing a survey of 193 Korean Americans between 50 and 75 years of age, they found that having CRC is positively associated with taking medical tours to the home country. According to their study, about one-third of Korean Americans in the greater Seattle area have experienced at least one medical tour to Korea. Those who were uninsured, who came to the United States when they were older, who stayed in the United States for a shorter period, who had received higher education, who did not have a "usual place of care," and who did not speak English well were more likely to take medical tours to the home country than their counterparts. Although their survey respondents were restricted to Korean Americans at least 50 years of age, their study is useful in that it served to illustrate a frequency of medical tourism and associated factors in one particular region in the United States.

## A REVIEW OF LITERATURE ON KOREAN IMMIGRANTS' HEALTHCARE BEHAVIORS

### Barriers to US Healthcare Utilization

Although Korean Americans have been praised as a "model minority" due to their higher educational attainment than the general population in the United States, most studies of Korean immigrants' healthcare behaviors have found that they also face various barriers and difficulties in access to the formal healthcare system in the United States (Choi 2013; De Gagne et al. 2014; Jang, Kim, and Chiriboga 2005; Ryu, Young, and Park 2001; Shin 2002; Song et al. 2010). As indicated in Introduction, immigrants' barriers to healthcare can be placed into three categories: structural, financial, and personal barriers.

In examining Korean immigrants' healthcare utilization, researchers have focused on financial or personal barriers rather than structural barriers for several reasons. First, since Korean immigrants include a much smaller proportion of illegal residents than Latino or Filipino immigrants (Hoefer, Rytina, and Baker 2009), researchers have not paid much attention to Koreans' legal status as a structural barrier to the US healthcare system. Moreover, since Korean immigrants are concentrated in several metropolitan areas (Min 2013), they are less likely to have transportation issues associated with visiting doctor's offices or hospitals than other immigrant groups that are residentially more scattered.

Thus, researchers of Korean immigrants' healthcare behaviors have instead focused on their financial barriers, especially their health insurance status, in order to investigate their healthcare patterns (Jang, Kim, and Chiriboga 2005; Ryu, Young, and Park 2001; Shin et al. 2005). In fact, Korean immigrants show a very low insurance rate compared to other major Asian immigrant groups. Analyzing the 1998 Current Population Survey (CPS), Carrasquillo et al. (2000) found that more than one-third of Korean immigrants do not have public health insurance, while only 58% of Korean immigrants have private health insurance. Among all major Asian immigrant groups, only Vietnamese immigrants show a lower rate of private health insurance (50%) than Korean immigrants. Chinese (69%), Indian (76%), and Filipino (70%) immigrant groups show much higher private health insurance rates than Korean immigrants.

Using national data, Ryu, Young, and Park (2001) compared Korean Americans and other Asian-American groups in terms of their rates of health insurance. The results of their analysis of the 1992 NHIS indicated that Korean Americans show a much lower insurance rate (50%) compared to all Asian ethnic groups (70%). They also emphasized three additional significant results. First, health insurance is a significant predictor of better healthcare utilization among Korean Americans. Second, the impact of health insurance on healthcare utilization is greater for Korean Americans than for Asian-Americans in general. Lastly, self-employed Koreans are the least likely to be insured.

Previous research has found that Korean immigrants' low health insurance is related to their high concentration of entrepreneurship or ethnic business in the United States, where one's health insurance is highly influenced by one's employment status. Since the vast majority of Korean immigrants are self-employed in small businesses or are employed in small Korean firms, they have a lower rate of health insurance than other Asian groups (Ryu, Young, and Park 2001; You and Kim 2008). Among Korean immigrants, self-employed Koreans show a lower rate of health insurance than Koreans who work in the public sector or non-ethnic private sector (Ryu, Young, and Park 2001). Korean immigrants in the United States with no health insurance have great difficulties obtaining healthcare, and their distress in this situation is likely to be compounded by the fact that they would have been protected by the national healthcare system provided by the Korean government before their immigration to the United Stated. Later in this chapter, the differences in health insurance rates by Korean immigrants' self-employment status are compared by analyzing the ACS data. Later in chapter 4, I will analyze my own data to examine whether self-employed Korean immigrants show a higher rate of underutilization in the United States and a higher rate of taking medical tours to Korea to overcome this financial barrier.

Unlike insured status, which shows more evident and consistent findings, the influence of Korean immigrants' personal barriers is often insignificant or inconsistent across different studies. For example, regarding the language barrier, some studies have found a positive association between English proficiency and Koreans' healthcare utilization in the United States (De Gagne et al. 2014; Juon, Choi, and Kim 2000). By contrast, another study found that English proficiency was not a statistically significant factor in Koreans' hospital visits (Jang, Kim, and Chiriboga 2005). The association between acculturation and healthcare utilization also seems to be contradictory. De Gagne et al. (2014) found a positive association between middle-aged Korean immigrants' acculturation (measured by the length of time spent in the United States) and healthcare utilization. However, other studies indicated that the number of years in the United States was not a statistically significant factor to elderly Korean immigrants' healthcare utilization in LA (Sohn and Harada 2014). It is likely that, due to the many Korean social service agencies and elderly centers in LA, new Korean immigrants might have less difficulty in getting access to the US healthcare system compared to those in other smaller Korean communities.

## Korean Immigrants' Coping Strategies against Barriers to Formal US Healthcare

As briefly pointed out in Introduction, immigrants display several behavioral strategies to cope with the aforementioned structural, financial, and personal barriers to formal US healthcare. As indicated earlier, some Korean immigrants go back to the home country for medical care when they face barriers to formal healthcare in the United States. (Since their medical tourism behaviors were reviewed earlier, the discussion will not be repeated here.) Going to free clinics or community health centers has been used as a coping strategy among immigrants in general, especially undocumented or uninsured immigrants, because these clinics offer free (albeit limited) medical care without asking about patients' legal status or insured status (Kamimura et al. 2013; Okie 2007; Portes, Fernández-Kelly, and Light 2012). However, Korean community centers in the NY-NJ area do not offer any health treatments due to liability issues, so Korean immigrants in this area do not have the opportunity to go to free clinics supported by the ethnic community.

Seeing co-ethnic doctors is one of the coping strategies that Korean immigrants can utilize in practice. Despite the small number of co-ethnic doctors, immigrants still prefer and seek co-ethnic doctors because of language barriers, cultural differences, and their limited knowledge of Western medicine (Choi 2013; Wang 2007; Wang, Rosenberg, and Lo 2008; Zhang and Verhoef 2002). In particular, Asian-Americans with limited English proficiency are more likely to see co-racial doctors (LaVeist and Nuru-Jeter 2002). Previous studies reveal that Korean immigrants also prefer Korean doctors due to language barriers and communication issues with non-Korean-speaking doctors. For example, slightly more than a quarter of middle-aged Korean immigrants in North Carolina are not able to communicate in English with others. Thus, they prefer to see Korean health professionals (De Gagne et al. 2014). Another study (Son 2013) showed that about 30% of female Korean immigrants in Wisconsin do not understand well what non-Korean doctors say.

In addition to language barriers, health insurance status is also related to Korean immigrants' preference for co-ethnic doctors. Choi (2013) indicated that Korean immigrants often experience a radical change in health insurance status after their migration to the United States. Unlike Korea, which offers a national health insurance program for all citizens, the US health insurance is closely related to the individual's employment status. As will be shown in detail later in this chapter, Korean immigrants show a high proportion of self-employment; thus, they tend not to have health insurance. Therefore, they are likely to try to seek healthcare in their ethnic community and are more likely to choose co-ethnic doctors over non-co-ethnic doctors.

Using complementary and alternative medicine (CAM) is another coping behavior among immigrants, including Koreans. Previous studies have shown that immigrants who have barriers to formal healthcare are more likely to use CAM (Akresh 2009; Han 2001; Hill et al. 2006; Kim and Chan 2004; Portes, Fernández-Kelly, and Light 2012; Pourat et al. 1999; Wu, Burke, and LeBaron 2007). Korean immigrants' practice of a non-Western form of Korean traditional medicine has been referred to by various names, such as CAM, traditional medicine, oriental medicine, or folk medicine. Han (1997 and 2001) calls it *Hanbang*, which comprises both herbal medicine and acupuncture, and which can be used for both preventive and treatment purposes. He also defines it as a traditional medicine that "originated in China and indigenized in Korea." In this book, I will refer to this type of medicine as *Hanbang* because this is how it is called by most people in Korea and how it appears in the newspaper articles related to medical tourism.

Hill et al. (2006) found that a significant proportion of Korean immigrants use *Hanbang* as one of their healthcare options; about a quarter of Korean immigrants in California, as well as Koreans in Korea, use traditional medicine. Although many Korean immigrants utilize *Hanbang*, only a few solely depend on it. According to Kim et al. (2002), 3.9% of elderly Korean immigrants in the Baltimore area utilize only Korean traditional medicine, whereas more than half of them utilize only Western medicine. These findings suggest that many Korean immigrants mainly depend on Western medicine as their primary form of medical treatment while using *Hanbang* as alternative medicine only occasionally. In fact, scholars have found that Korean immigrants consider *Hanbang* to be a supplementary treatment, rather than the main treatment, for their healthcare (Choi 2013; Kim et al. 2002).

There are several factors associated with Korean immigrants' practice of *Hanbang*. First, the level of acculturation is associated with it, but the direction of this association differs across various studies. For example, using multiple logistic regression analysis, Kim and Chan (2004) found a high level of education, a high degree of acculturation to the US society and a shorter period of stay in the United States to be positively associated with Korean immigrants' preference for alternative medicine. Their findings are congruent with the earlier findings by Miller (1990), who showed that more educated and more acculturated Korean immigrants have a greater tendency to seek alternative medicine. By contrast, Hill et al. (2006) discovered that less acculturated Korean immigrants are more likely to see a traditional healer than are their more acculturated counterparts.

Health insurance is also associated with Korean immigrants' use of *Hanbang*. Like acculturation, health insurance status is both positively and negatively correlated with *Hanbang* in different studies. On the one hand, having health insurance is positively associated with visiting "traditional healers" among elderly Koreans in LA (Pourat et al. 1999). On the other hand, uninsured Korean Americans in California show a higher prevalence of seeing a "traditional practitioner" than their insured counterparts (Hill et al. 2006). The size of social network, better mental health status (Pourat et al. 1999), and the type of occupation (Han 2000) have also contributed to the practice of *Hanbang*. In Sydney, Australia, Han (2000) argued that Korean immigrants whose job requires physical movement tend to prefer alternative medicine compared to skilled migrants or businessmen.

## BACKGROUND INFORMATION ABOUT KOREAN IMMIGRANTS IN THE UNITED STATES

### Demographic and Socioeconomic Characteristics

Table 1.1 compares the demographic characteristics of foreign-born Koreans with those of native-born Koreans and native-born whites in the United States. There are substantially more female than male Korean immigrants, whereas gender is more balanced among native-born Koreans and native-born whites. About 60% of Korean immigrants are female compared to 52% of their native-born Koreans and white counterparts. On average, Korean immigrants are slightly younger (47 years old) than non-Hispanic whites (51 years old), but older than native-born Koreans (29 years old) when only adult respondents are included in the analysis. Numbers in Table 1.1 show that Korean immigrants are younger than native-born whites but much older than native-born Koreans: about 15% of Korean immigrants are elderly (65 years old and older) compared to 19% of native-born whites and only 1.3% of native-born Koreans. As Appendix presents, the gender and age distributions of the 507 survey respondents used for this book are very similar to those of all Korean immigrants in the United States, as quota sampling has been applied to collect the survey data; about 55.8% of survey respondents are female, and 17% of them are elderly.

The post-1965 immigration cohort has a high level of education. Also, as earlier scholars have pointed out, they had white-collar occupations with a middle-class urban background prior to their migration to the United States (Kim 1981; Min 1988, 2005 and 2013; Yoon 1991). Table 1.1 supports these

**Table 1.1 Characteristics by Country of Birth and Ethnicity (%)**

| | *Foreign-born Koreans* | *Native-born Koreans* | *Native-born Whites* |
|---|---|---|---|
| Demographic Characteristics | | | |
| Female | 59.4 | 52.6 | 51.9 |
| Mean age | 46.6 | 29.3 | 50.7 |
| Elderly (65 years old and older)[1] | 14.5 | 1.3 | 19.1 |
| Post-1965 immigration cohort | 97.8 | – | 73.9 |
| Naturalized citizen | 59.6 | – | – |
| *N* | 25,268 | 3,839 | 4,866,205 |
| Socioeconomic Characteristics | | | |
| Educational Level | | | |
| High school graduates | 91.0 | 98.3 | 90.6 |
| College graduates | 52.4 | 71.7 | 30.5 |
| *N* (25 years old and older) | 22,894 | 2,187 | 4,388,241 |
| Occupational Characteristics | | | |
| Management and professional occupations[2] | 49.2 | 66.7 | 43.2 |
| Mean wage and salary income ($) | 50,157 | 68,595 | 50,557 |
| *N* (25–64 years old and currently employed) | 12,439 | 1,624 | 2,350,749 |
| Self-employed[3] | 24.3 | 8.4 | 11.5 |
| *N* (25–64 years old and in the labor market) | 13,334 | 1,752 | 2,528,633 |

[1]The analysis for the percentage of elderly includes all respondents (*N* of all foreign-born Koreans: 27,810; *N* of all native-born Koreans: 8,237; *N* of all native-born non-Hispanic whites: 6,059,816).

[2]The analysis of the management/professional occupations and the mean of wage and salary income include respondents who are 25–64 years old and currently employed (*N* of foreign-born Korean: 12,439; *N* of native-born Korean: 1,624; *N* of native-born white: 2,350,749).

[3]The analysis of self-employment includes respondents who are 25–64 years old and participate in the labor market (*N* of foreign-born Korean: 13,334; *N* of native-born Korean: 1,752; *N* of native-born white: 2,528,633).

*Source*: The ACS (2009–2011).

earlier findings. The vast majority of foreign-born Koreans (91%) are high school graduates, and more than half of them (52.4%) are college graduates. Their high school and college completion rates are higher than those of native-born whites but lower than those of native-born Koreans. Although the variation in the educational level is not great among Korean immigrants, an earlier study (Ko et al. 2016) found that higher educational level is associated with Korean immigrants' engagement in medical tours to the home country; thus, in chapter 4, I examine whether education is one of contributing factors to Korean immigrants' medical tourism, because the level of education could be a mediating factor to other contributing factors. In this investigation, I seek to answer the following questions: Would more educated Koreans show a higher rate of medical tourism than less educated Koreans because they have more transnational ties with the home country through their alumni associations? Alternatively, would they show a lower rate of medical tourism because they have more social networks in the United States through their high human capital?

Korean immigrants show higher rates of managerial and professional occupations than native-born whites. Nearly half of them have managerial and professional occupations. As expected, native-born Koreans show even higher representation (66.7%) in these two occupational categories than do foreign-born Koreans (49.2%). Korean immigrants show a slightly lower mean wage and salary income ($50,157) than native-born whites ($50,557), despite their higher engagement in managerial and professional jobs. Disadvantages in the US labor market, especially the language barrier, are the major contributing factors to Korean immigrants' higher self-employment rates compared to native-born whites and other Asian immigrant subgroups (Min 1984, 1990 and 2008; Min and Bozorgmehr 2003; Yoon 1991). Confirming previous studies, Table 1.1 shows that nearly a quarter of Korean immigrants are self-employed, whereas only 8.4% of native-born Koreans and 11.5% of native-born whites are self-employed. It should be noted that the national statistical data underestimate the numbers of Korean immigrant entrepreneurs, because most small Korean businesses are run by a family, usually a husband and a wife, and in such cases, only the husband tends to be the registered owner when they respond to national surveys (Min 2013).

Table 1.2 shows that, in general, Korean immigrants have a much lower health insurance rate (74.4%) than native-born non-Hispanic whites (89.4%) or other major foreign-born Asian groups. Having a much higher self-employment rate than other Asian immigrant groups is one of the reasons for Korean immigrants' lower insurance rates compared to other Asian immigrant groups. In fact, self-employed Korean immigrants are less likely to be insured (60.1%) than employed Korean immigrants (88.7%) and other self-employed immigrant groups. Moreover, there are two other reasons besides the higher self-employment rate for Korean immigrants' lower insurance rates compared to other Asian immigrant groups. First, unlike Korean immigrants, who tend to work in labor-intensive small businesses, Indian and Filipino immigrants tend to own and work in professional businesses, such as health or finance fields. Thus, they are more likely to have better benefits, including health insurance. Second, they have higher rates of working in American corporations compared to Korean immigrants. Unlike Koreans who have their own businesses or who work in the ethnic economy, other immigrants who work in American corporations get better health insurance coverage.

Due to their uninsured status, self-employed Korean immigrants might have a greater tendency to take medical tours to the home country. Alternatively, rather than their uninsured status, their long working hours as entrepreneurs

**Table 1.2 Health Insurance Rate by Self-Employment Status (%)**

| | *Foreign-born Korean* | *Foreign-born Chinese* | *Foreign-born Indian* | *Foreign-born Filipino* | *Foreign-born Vietnamese* | *US-born Non-Hispanic White* |
|---|---|---|---|---|---|---|
| Self-employed | 60.1 | 75.5 | 79.1 | 78.4 | 66.3 | 82.9 |
| Employed | 88.7 | 89.9 | 98.3 | 99.2 | 91.9 | 95.9 |
| All | 74.4 | 82.7 | 88.7 | 88.8 | 79.1 | 89.4 |
| Total *N*[1] | 25,268 | 2,784 | 43,600 | 43,303 | 26,594 | 5,114,091 |

[1]Adult (18 years old or older) respondents who had worked within the past 5 years are included in this analysis.
*Note*: Except for US-born white, all other categories include foreign-born, non-Hispanic individuals who consider themselves to be Asian.
*Source*: The ACS (2009–2011).

might be a mediating factor in the association between self-employment and medical tourism. In chapter 4, Korean immigrants' self-employment status, along with other sociodemographic characteristics, will be examined to determine whether these factors are associated with their decision to engage in medical tourism.

## Strong Ethnic Attachment

Another distinctive characteristic of Korean immigrants is that they show a higher degree of ethnic attachment and a lower level of assimilation compared to other Asian immigrant groups. For example, Min (1991, 1998) has shown that Korean immigrants maintain a higher level of ethnic attachment than other Asian immigrant groups. He discussed three major contributing factors to Korean immigrants' ethnic attachments: the degree of group homogeneity, the degree of religious affiliation and practices, and their economic segregation.

First, Korean immigrants are much more culturally homogenous than other Asian immigrant groups. Korean immigrants have one language, compared to other Asian immigrant groups that have several different languages. Also, Korean immigrants have a much lower level of regional differences than Chinese, Indian, or Filipino immigrants, as more than half of them lived in Seoul prior to their migration, and three-quarters of them are from the five largest cities in Korea (Park et al. 1990; Min 1996). In addition, Korean immigrants have a higher level of class homogeneity than Chinese immigrants (Kwong 1997).

Second, about 75% of Korean immigrants are Christians, and an overwhelming majority of them participate in ethnic churches with great frequency (Hurh and Kim 1990; Min 1992; Min and Jang 2015). Researchers have found that religion is a significant source of Korean immigrants' ethnic attachment because religious activities based on ethnic congregations can help them maintain their cultural traditions and social networks (Hurh and Kim 1990; Min 2001; Pang 1991). Pang (1991) pointed out that Korean ethnic churches provide social supports for elderly Korean immigrants. Min (2001) found that there are about 600 Korean ethnic churches in the New York metropolitan area, which help Korean immigrants maintain ethnic traditions and ethnic networks.

Lastly, as pointed out earlier, Korean immigrants show much higher self-employment rates than native-born whites and other immigrant groups, which further socially isolate them within the ethnic community. Moreover, as a response to conflicts with white suppliers and Black customers, Korean immigrants in New York City use ethnic collective actions far more frequently than other immigrant groups (Min 1996, 2008). The Korean Produce Association (KPA) based in the NY-NJ area helps them to maintain strong ethnic attachments by supporting Korean entrepreneurs and providing networks for Korean immigrants. The KPA has annually organized the Korean Harvest and Folklore Festival since 1982 to celebrate *Chuseok* (Korean Thanksgiving Day) together, to transmit Korean folk culture to younger-generation Koreans, and to promote Korean cultural traditions to New Yorkers (Min 2008).

Other types of associations, alumni associations, social service agencies, business associations, and political organizations have also played important roles in providing Korean immigrants with ethnic networks and social services (Min 2001). For example, the Korean American Association of Greater New York (KAAGNY) has played a key role in organizing the Korean Parade in Manhattan annually since 1980 and preparing ceremonies for two important Korean national holidays, Independence Movement Day and Independence Day (Min 2008). In chapter 2, I examine how the KAAGNY has cooperated with Korean hospitals to attract more Korean immigrant medical tourists.

## Transnational Ties with the Home Country

Based on a survey in the NY-NJ area, Min (2013b) found strong social transnational ties with the home country among Korean immigrants; about 85% of Korean permanent residents and naturalized citizens have visited Korea since their migration to the United States. More than half of them (54%) have visited Korea three or more times. However, despite their frequent visits to Korea, the studies of Korean immigrants' transnationalism in the United States and Canada are scarce (Kwak and Hiebert 2010).

As indicated in the theory section of Introduction, researchers have classified immigrant transnationalism into several different fields: political, economic, social, cultural, and religious. Most studies of Korean immigrants' transnational ties to the homeland have focused on the social and cultural fields. Noh, Kwak, and Han (2013) measured the degree of Korean immigrants' social transnational ties by the number of relatives and friends they had in Korea and the frequency of their contact with them. They found strong social transnational ties among Korean immigrants in Canada, noting that more than half of them had at least one parent in Korea, and about 80% of them had talked to their relatives via telephone. They also concluded that social transnational ties are stronger for younger and more recent immigrants.

Recently, researchers have given much attention to Korean immigrants' cultural transnationalism. Min (2012) indicated two types of immigrants' cultural transnational activities: (1) consuming cultural content through the transnational media and (2) participating in cultural events organized by the home country. Other scholars (Noh, Kwak, and Han 2013) have found strong cultural transnationalism of the first type: more than 80% of their Korean respondents in Toronto watched Korean TV programs, read Korean newspaper or magazines, and connected to Korean websites on a daily basis. Regarding the second type of cultural transnationalism, Min (2012) conducted a content analysis using newspaper articles published by two Korean dailies in the NY-NJ area in 2010. He categorized transnational cultural events into five groups: performing arts, fine arts, food-related events, language and literature, and others. He found that performing arts (e.g., music, dances, musicals, and plays) were the most frequent types of transnational cultural events among Korean immigrants.

Compared to their social and cultural transnationalism, Korean immigrants' political, economic, and religious transnationalism are under-researched. This is probably due to their low participation in transnational activities in these fields. Noh and his associates (2013) found that Korean immigrants are not very active in political transnational activities: 3.3% of their respondents participated in the Korean election and only 1% of them participated in a Korean political organization. On the other hand, their Korean immigrant respondents showed stronger economic transnational ties with the home country; more than 60% of them sent or received money or gifts to or from Korea. Moreover, about 70% of them maintained their economic assets in Korea even after their migration. Although Korean immigrants show minimal political, economic, and religious transnational activities, the association between other types of transnationalism and medical transnationalism will be examined in chapter 4.

Recently, researchers have examined one particular type of Korean transnational family: a *Kirogi* (wild goose) family. This type of transnational family is composed of a mother and children living in the United States for the children's education while the father stays in Korea to support the family financially (Ahn 2009; Cha 2010; Jeong, You, and Kwon 2013; Kang 2012;

Kim 2009; Lee 2010; Song 2010; Song 2012). The *Kirogi* family is so called because wild geese mate for life, and if one of the pair dies the other dedicates him- or herself to raising the offspring alone. This situation resembles a transnational *Kirogi* family, in which the mother who devotes herself to raising children alone in a foreign country. I hypothesized that the members of a *Kirogi* family would have a stronger transnational tie with the home country (compared to Korean immigrants who have all their family members in the Unites States) and, thus, would be more likely to take medical tours to the home country. This hypothesis will be discussed in chapter 4.

As pointed out earlier, Korean immigrants' medical transnationalism and medical tourism to the home country also have not received much attention from scholars. This is partly due to the recency of the popularity of the medical tourism phenomenon in Korea, as will be explained in chapter 2. It is also partly due to the lack of data on Korean immigrants' medical tourism and other medical transnational activities with the home country. This book, which examines Korean immigrants' medical tourism using both quantitative and qualitative data, is intended to help fill this gap in the literature on immigrant medical transnationalism.

*Chapter 2*

# The Development of Medical Tourism in Korea and the Related Issues

## MEDICAL TOURISM IN COMPETING ASIAN COUNTRIES

The development of medical tourism can bring in foreign currency, create more medical jobs, produce more tax revenue, and expand the health industry of a country (Bookman and Bookman 2007; De Arellano 2007; Garcia-Altes 2005; Lunt and Carrera 2010; Reddy et al. 2010). In addition to the economic reasons, medical tourism can contribute to the destination countries by preventing a brain drain of doctors and nurses, allowing them to remain in their country of origin (De Arellano 2007). Thus, as an active entity of *state transnationalism*, several destination countries actively promote medical tourism in their own countries for their national interests.

Korea and three other competing Asian countries (India, Singapore, and Thailand), the top three medical tourism destination countries who are about to take charge of more than 80% market share in Asia (Mary 2014; Ganguli and Ebrahim 2017), have shown different characteristics of medical tourism and strategies to attract more medical tourists. Foreign patients who visit these four countries come from all over the world. However, patients from the United States comprised a high proportion of the total number of foreign patients from India, Thailand, and Korea (Chinai and Goswami 2007; Tawichai and Antaseeda 2002). Singapore receives patients mostly from its neighbors: Indonesia, Malaysia, Bangladesh, and Vietnam (International Medical Travel Journal 2013). Each country has its own specialization in medical treatments. For example, India and Singapore seem to specialize in cardiac surgery, knee or hip replacement surgery, and cancer treatments. Thailand is known for its postoperative care, spa, massage, alternative therapies, and tropical climate (Harryono et al. 2006). Foreign patients in Korea also go for elective care, such as regular checkups, cosmetic surgery, or skin treatments.

Each country seems to have its own strengths of medical tourism. For example, the medical cost of India is less expensive than the United States and even less expensive than other Asian countries, such as Thailand and Singapore (Dawn and Pal 2011). Thailand also invites foreign patients for cheaper medical costs and warm tropical climate for relaxation. Singapore seems to appeal to patients who speak English (Singapore's official language) and who are impressed by the quality of the country's medical services and professionals. As An (2014) pointed out, one of Korea's advantages in bringing in more foreign patients is *Hallyu*, the worldwide popularity of Korean culture, an example of cultural globalization. How the Korean government and private sector agencies utilize *Hallyu* to promote medical tourism will be discussed in detail later in this chapter.

Each government has its own strategy to promote medical tourism. Although there is no national organization that supports medical tourism (Moghavvemi et al. 2017), the government of India issues two special medical tourism visas to foreign patients (De Arellano 2007; Reddy et al. 2010; Reed 2008): (1) the Tourist Visa on Arrival (TVOA) for a short-term medical tour and (2) a medical visa for a long-term one. Applicants from any eligible country can apply, pay for, and receive the TVOA online and stay in India for up to 30 days. Moreover, foreign tourists with a medical visa can stay in India for up to one year, which is longer than for holders of a regular tourist visa. The recipient of the medical visa can also leave and reenter India up to three times in that year.

Like the government of India, the Thai government has streamlined the visa process for foreign patients; the individuals who want to visit Thailand for the medical purpose can stay up to 90 days with nonimmigrant visa (Wong et al. 2014). Besides, Thai government's "Amazing Thailand" campaign promotes the country's excellent spas, hospitals, and herbal products (Teh 2007). The Thai government has set a governmental guideline and standard for spas and massages that specialize in spa medical tourism (Hurh et al. 2013).

The government of Singapore, another famous medical tourism country, seems to be the most active among these four Asian medical tourism destination countries. It has established a national initiative, "Singapore Medicine," to make Singapore the hub of medical care in Asia (Hurh et al. 2013). This "government-industry partnership" has been created for medical tourists as well as various issues related to medical tourism, such as medical research, medical education, medical conferences, and exhibitions (Ganguli and Ebrahim 2017). Three government organizations promote medical tourism in Singapore: the Singapore Tourism Board (STB), the Economic Development Board (EDB), and the International Enterprise Singapore (IES). The STB takes charge of marketing and branding (Ganguli and Ebrahim 2017), contacts medical tourism organizations in other countries, develops medical tourism programs, and induces collaborative programs between hospitals and travel agencies (Lee and

Park 2013). The EDB supports medical tourism through investment and industrial growth in the medical industry. IES supports health professionals' overseas activities. The Korean government's strategies to promote medical tourism will be detailed in the following section of this chapter.

## THE DEVELOPMENT OF MEDICAL TOURISM AND THE KOREAN GOVERNMENT'S EFFORTS TO PROMOTE IT

Lower medical costs comprise one of the strongest factors that contribute to medical tourism to Korea. For example, Koechlin, Lorenzoni, and Schreyer (2010) compared the price levels of hospital services among 12 countries who joined the OECD. The United States ranked the first in the price level in various hospital services, whereas Korea had the lowest price level. The United States has about three times as high as the price level of inpatient hospital services and about 10 times as high prices of inpatient surgery as Korea. When it comes to real medical costs rather than the price level, Korea still shows significantly cheaper medical expenses for various surgeries and hospital services than other OECD countries. For example, in 2007, a knee replacement surgery cost US$14,946 in the United States, but only US$9,222 in Korea (OECD 2011). Dental treatments showed the greatest disparity; dental costs in the United States were 15 to 25 times higher than in Korea (Ryu et al. 2015).

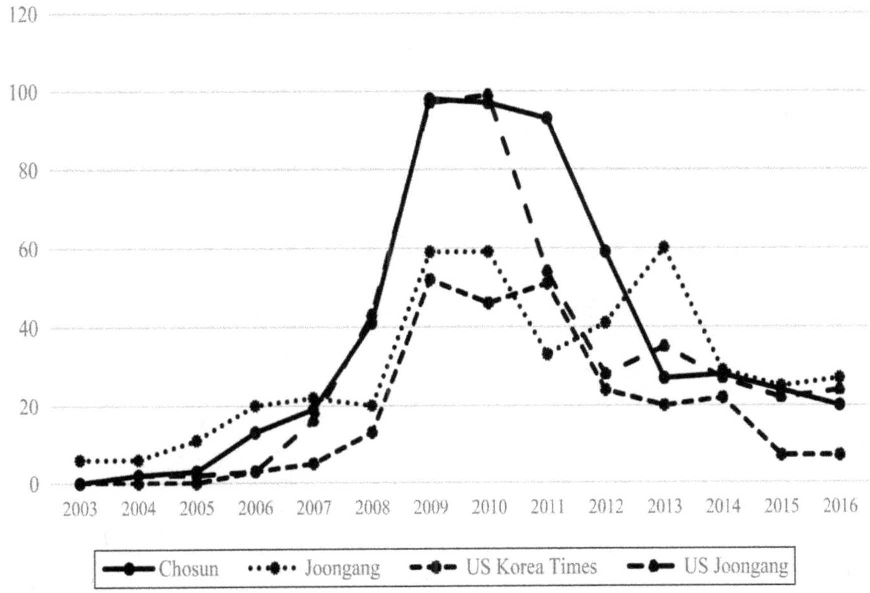


**Figure 2.1 Changes in the Numbers of Medical Tourism Articles by Year and Daily Newspaper.**

With the advantage of cheaper medical expenses, the Korean government has put efforts to develop medical tourism in Korea. Figure 2.1 shows the trend of medical tourism in Korea by presenting the changes in the quantity of articles published in four Korean newspapers for over 10 years (January 1, 2003, to December 31, 2016) using the keyword *medical tourism*. It suggests three phases of medical tourism in Korea: pioneering (2005–2008), prosperity (2009–2011), and stagnation (2012–2016).

As Figure 2.1 shows, the number of articles about medical tourism was negligible before 2005. However, as Table 2.1 also presents, 2005 was the pioneer

**Table 2.1 The Korean Government's Various Efforts to Promote Medical Tourism**

| *Year* | *Contents* |
|---|---|
| 2005 | • Added medical tourism to the official governmental agenda |
| 2006 | • Implemented research on expansion of global medical services and foreign patients |
| 2007 | • Secured budget to attract foreign patients<br>• Established the Korea International Medical Association (KIMA) to support medical tourism |
| 2009 | • Revised the medical law: introducing, arranging, and inviting foreign patients became legal<br>• Enforced the registration system of promotion agencies that attract foreign patients<br>• Issued a medical visa (M visa) to foreign patients<br>• Established the Medical Tourism One-stop Service Center for foreign patients<br>• Developed the Korean medical brand, "Smart Care, Medical Korea"<br>• Trained medical tourism coordinators and translators specialized in medical tourism |
| 2010 | • Introduced an authentication system of medical institutions<br>• Revised the medical law: the medical institutions that intend to attract foreign patients should be registered with the Korean government |
| 2011 | • Enhanced the "Two Stage Enhancement Plan for Medical Tourism"<br>• Applied a temporary zero tax rate (for 2011 and 2012) for commission among companies who do business with medical institutions<br>• Signed the Memorandum of Understanding (MOU) with UAE, Dubai, and Mongolia<br>• Relaxed regulation on E-7 visa (Special Occupations) for foreign medical professionals and foreign medical tourism coordinators |
| 2012 | • Enhanced the "Plan for Vitalization Global Healthcare"<br>• Established the Medical Korea Academy Center<br>• Introduced medical tourism translation services |
| 2013 | • Enacted the revised electronic visa system<br>• Noticed an advanced legislation of Medi-tel (Medicine+Hotel)<br>• Established a national skill qualification certificate on international medical tourism coordinators |

*Source*: Statistics on International Patients in Korea (KHIDI 2013).

year of medical tourism in Korea; the Korean government placed medical tourism on the national agenda for the first time, and medical tourism in Korea has been developed since then with the government's efforts to promote it. In 2006, the Korean government began to conduct research on medical tourism to attract foreign patients. In 2007, it secured a budget for foreign patients and established the Korea International Medical Association (KIMA) to publicize Korean medical institutions and to provide information about medical tourism to foreign patients. These efforts were not as aggressive as they would become. The newspaper articles published in this pioneering period reported on countries like India, Malaysia, and Singapore which successfully promoted medical tourism so that the Korean government could emulate them.

It should be emphasized that the year of 2009 was a monumental year for medical tourism in Korea, beginning the prosperity period (2009–2011). As previous study (Jun and Oh 2015) confirmed, the number of newspaper articles about medical tourism surged between 2009 and 2011. Since 2009, the Korean government, as an active entity of state transnationalism, has promoted medical tourism with great enthusiasm. The Korean government revised the medical law to legalize inviting and arranging for foreign patients. After the revision of the 2009 medical law, the Korean government strengthened the basis to attract foreign patients and to develop the medical tourism industry. For example, all private agencies which dealt with foreign patients were required to register with the government. The medical visa was issued so that foreign patients could come and stay in Korea more easily. The Korean government opened the Medical Tourism One-Stop Service Center at the Incheon airport to assist foreign patients. Moreover, a Korean medical brand was designed, with a slogan, "Smart Care, Medical Korea," and a website (www.medicalkorea.or.kr) to give medical tourism information to foreign patients. Lastly, the Korean government introduced training programs for medical tourism coordinators and translators.

Since 2010, the Korean government has continued to encourage the growth and promotion of the medical tourism industry. For example, the authentication system of medical institutions made it much easier for foreign patients to find registered medical institutions in Korea. Since 2011, the Korean government has built a global network to promote medical tourism through Memorandums of Understanding (MOUs) with the United Arab Emirates (UAE), Dubai, and Mongolia. It also enacted a law to resolve medical conflicts between patients and medical institutions through the Korea Medical Dispute Mediation and Arbitration Agency. For two years the Korean government applied a zero tax rate to corporations that conducted business with medical institutions. It also relaxed regulations on E-7 visas for special occupations so that foreign healthcare professionals and medical tourism coordinators could obtain visas.

While the Korean government opened the door to foreign patients during the prosperity period, it continued to enhance plans for the diversification of medical tourism during the stagnation period. In 2012, it began to invite foreign patients from Saudi Arabia, Qatar, Iraq, Kazakhstan, Uzbekistan, Vietnam, Indonesia, and Russia. Unlike the United States, China, and Japan, these countries had no history of sending patients to Korea. In 2012, the Korean government began to provide translation services to foreign patients so that they could consult with staff at the Korean Medical Dispute Mediation and Arbitration Agency. Translation services were offered in 18 languages, including English, Chinese, Japanese, Vietnamese, Russian, German, and Spanish.

In 2013, the Korean government revised its electronic visa system, which allowed foreign patients to obtain Korean visas online. Moreover, it announced Medi-tel legislation (a Medi-tel combines a medical institution and a hotel). Lastly, the Korean government began to require prospective international medical tourism coordinators to pass a national examination, which assumed a knowledge of public health, tourism, marketing, and medical terminology.

Despite the Korean government's efforts, the number of articles about medical tourism began to decline in 2011. In 2011, more than 200 articles about Korean medical tourism were published, but the number had dropped to 140 by 2013 and to 78 by 2016. One possible reason is that medical tourism had been exhaustively covered during the prosperity period (2009–2011) and it had been stabilized after that. Notably, during the stagnation period, articles about problems with medical tourism started appearing. The later section will explore some of these issues, such as inconsistencies in medical tourism terminology by different governmental departments and brokerage problems.

Besides the Korean government, several local governments have developed specialized medical tourism programs that represented their cities. Noticeably, in conjunction with the increasing global popularity of *Hallyu*, also known as the *Korean Wave*, several local governments have tried to attract foreign patients to their cities, connecting *Hallyu* to cosmetic surgery. Gangnam-gu in Seoul and Seomyeon in Busan are the two main neighborhoods in Korea's two largest cities that actively attracted Chinese and Japanese patients who want to look like *Hallyu* stars for cosmetic surgery and skin treatments. For them, the before-and-after photos of their favorite Korean *Hallyu* star draw them to Korea for cosmetic surgery (Lee 2010). Gangnam-gu, one of the wealthiest districts in Korea, had 342 cosmetic surgery hospitals, about 72% of all cosmetic surgery hospitals in Seoul. To attract more foreign patients who were interested in cosmetic surgery, it has hosted an annual medical tourism roadshow since 2009 (Sohn 2012) to attract Japanese and Chinese patients who enjoy *Hallyu*. Gangnam-gu established a medical tourism team and selected 30 translators who could translate Japanese, Chinese, and Thai to support hospitals located in there (Kim 2009). Moreover, Gangnam-gu was the first district of Seoul to offer its own medical tourism package program to treat foreign cosmetic surgery patients to the shops, restaurants, or hair salons that Korean *Hallyu* stars have visited (Kang 2013; Lee 2010). Unlike other local governments that use *Hallyu* to attract foreign patients, this package features the "everyday life" of *Hallyu stars*. In other words, they not only target foreign patients those who want to "look" like *Hallyu stars* for cosmetic surgery or skin treatments but also those who want to live like them.

Seomyeon, located in the city of Busan, is another local government that tried to connect *Hallyu* and medical tourism. Busan, Korea's second largest city, established "Global Beauty Medical Streets" in Seomyeon to attract foreign patients who wanted to receive cosmetic surgery, skin treatments, dental care, and *Hanbang* care. There were more than 100 cosmetic surgery hospitals and skin care hospitals in Seomyeon. Given Busan's location on the southeastern coast of the Korean peninsula and its close geographic proximity to Japan, Japanese patients were the main target of medical tourism. To support medical tourism, the Busan city government established a call center to offer translation services to foreign patients who wanted to receive cosmetic surgery (Shim 2009).

## PRIVATE SECTOR AGENCIES' EFFORTS TO PROMOTE MEDICAL TOURISM

### Korean Hospitals

Among all private sector agencies, Korean hospitals were the most active in promoting medical tourism by offering foreign patients pickup services, translation services, and promotional events. Achieving Joint Commission International (JCI) accreditation was one notable strategy because the JCI was an internationally approved accreditation so that foreign patients could expect the guaranteed quality of the hospitals with the JCI. In addition to the JCI, some hospitals used distinct strategies to attract more foreign patients. One of them is Chaum Hospital, established in 2010 as a high-end medical institution with premium specialized services, such as the check-up center, the anti-aging center, the cell plastic surgery center, and the spa center. It offered star marketing (Ko 2010), which shows how cultural globalization was used to promote medical tourism in Korea. In 2010, Chaum invited about 120 international celebrities, including Kristin Davis, Peter Fonda, Sheena Easton, and Suzanne Somers. It was very unusual for foreign celebrities to come to Korea to promote medical treatments. Although Chaum's Hollywood star marketing and *Hallyu* marketing by Korean local governments are driven by cultural globalization and are closely connected to medical tourism, Chaum's strategy featured the hospital's trendsetting facilities and technologies whereas *Hallyu* marketing was used to appeal to Asian patients to want to look and live like Korean celebrities.

Another hospital, Cheongshim, specialized in the Japanese pregnant women's maternity trip (Chung 2011b). Although Cheongshim was not as big as Yonsei Severance and Samsung Hospital, it held the third rank in terms of attracting foreign patients in 2010. Concentrating on Japanese pregnant women was the key to its success. According to the interview with the staff at the hospital, it costs about US$7,300 for delivery of a baby if a Japanese pregnant woman stays for four nights and five days in a hospital in Japan. By contrast, it costs only about one-third if she stays for two weeks for childbirth as well as postpartum care in Cheongshim. As another strategy to attract Japanese pregnant women, the hospital helped to issue birth certificates and passports for the newborns of the Japanese mothers who came to give birth at the hospital.

Like some Korean local governments, several Korean hospitals, especially cosmetic surgery or dermatology hospitals, use *Hallyu* as a marketing strategy. In 2009, six cosmetic surgery specialists, dermatology offices, and dental offices worked together to publicize medical tourism programs in Tokyo, Japan (Kim 2009). At a medical tourism fair in Japan, the directors of six hospitals showed pictures of Korean *Hallyu* stars to Japanese patients to persuade them to undergo cosmetic surgery or skin treatments in Korea. They highlighted the importance of the combination of medical tourism and *Hallyu* because the medical services that they offered were closely related to *Hallyu*. In 2011, Dr. Lee, a director of Arumdaun Nara dermatology hospital, received an award from the Korean government to recognize his efforts to attract foreign patients to Korea. In 2011, more than 3,000 foreign patients visited his office to receive skin care. He emphasized the importance of linking *Hallyu* to medical tourism to attract more foreign patients to Korea (Kim 2011).

To investigate Korean hospitals' efforts and strategies to attract more foreign patients, I interviewed staff members at three big hospitals in Korea: Asan Medical Center, Yonsei Severance Hospital, and Inha University Hospital. They reported that the number of foreign patients had increased since 2009 after the revision of the medical law. Each hospital had its own strategy to attract foreign patients. For example, a staff member at Asan Medical Center described its strategy:

> Our foreign patients are mostly from the US, China, Japan, Russia, and UAE and we actively try to attract more of them since they spend a lot of money to

our medical center. On average, they spend US$10,000 for their medical treatments at our center. One interesting thing that we found was that some foreign patients visited our center to treat serious illness, such as cancer, and then they revisit our center with their family members for non-urgent medical care, such as cosmetic surgery or skin treatments. Since the number of patients from UAE is increasing, we recently signed a patient delivery contract with UAE and held promotional events at foreign embassies and international schools. Also, we invite doctors from Asian countries to provide them medical training so that patients from those countries can visit our center by referral from these doctors.

A staff member at Yonsei Severance Hospital mentioned that unlike Asan Medical Center, its patients, mostly from the United States, China, and Japan, visited their hospital for serious and acute illness. He emphasized the hospital's efforts to attract more foreign patients:

> On average, foreign patients spend US$9,000 to 13,000 for medical care at our hospital. To attract them to our hospital, we utilize various strategies, such as holding various events in the foreign countries to meet the future patients there, providing brochures about advantages of visiting our hospital to the foreign agencies so that they can distribute the booklets to future patients. Once they arrive in Korea, we provide them translation, transportation, and accommodation services so that they can stay in Korea more comfortable to focus on their medical treatments.

## Korean Travel Agencies

Compared to Korean hospitals, other private sector organizations were less engaged in attracting foreign patients to Korea. For instance, Hana Tour and Mode Tour are the two biggest travel agencies that promoted medical tourism. In 2008, Hana Tour developed its first medical tourism package in collaboration with Korea University Medical Center (Oh 2009). Mode Tour proposed a medical tourism package that targeted Chinese patients in cooperation with Gangnam-gu and Ana Clinic, a mega hospital that specialized in skin care. The Chinese patients who bought this package spent two days in Seoul for skin treatment and sightseeing and another two days in Jeju Island for sightseeing (Byun 2009). However, after 2009, no newspaper articles reported on any travel agencies' activity to attract foreign patients.

In addition to these two travel agencies, MeditourKorea was established in 2009. This new company specialized in medical tourism to Busan and marketed to Japanese patients. Meditour Korea also used *Hallyu* to promote medical tourism to Korea from Japan (Park 2009a). For example, it held a concert with the original soundtrack of *The Winter Sonata*, a Korean drama which played a significant role in promoting *Hallyu* in Japan.

### Korean Hotels

Korean hotels were the final type of private sector agency engaged in activities to attract more foreign patients. In 2013, Medi-tel, a specialized building for medical care and accommodation for foreign patients, was announced. However, the collaboration between hotels and hospitals began much earlier with a three-pronged strategy to promote medical tourism in Korea. First, some hotels gave a discount to guests who underwent medical care at an affiliated hotel. For example, Lotte City Hotel at Gimpo Airport and Wooridul Hospital signed an MOU so foreign patients who receive medical care at Wooridul Hospital could receive a discount at Lotte hotels (Suh et al. 2012). The second strategy was to invite hospitals or medical offices to share space in the building. By doing so, guests could receive medical care without leaving the hotel. This also protected the privacy of foreign patients. A Lotte Hotel in Busan invited the Korean Medical Institute to its hotel building so that foreign patients staying in the hotel could get on-site checkups (Park 2011). The last strategy was to construct a building that was half-hotel and half-hospital. In 2011, the first attempt was made to combine a hotel and a hospital to attract patients from foreign countries (Park 2011). In 2013, the legislation that allowed the establishment of Medi-tel opened a new phase of the medical tourism industry in Korea.

## THE EFFORTS TO PROMOTE KOREAN IMMIGRANTS' MEDICAL TOURISM

### The Korean Government

As already pointed out in Introduction, the Korean government does not define Korean immigrants with the US permanent residency as foreign patients. Nevertheless, it has made great efforts to bring overseas Koreans back to their home country to get medical care. The Korean government's efforts to attract Korean immigrant medical tourists can be considered as state transnationalism because their efforts are highly institutionalized. For example, in order to target Korean immigrants, the Korean government conducted several surveys with Korean immigrants. In 2006, the Korean Ministry of Health and Welfare published a report based on its survey of 271 Korean immigrants who lived in Pennsylvania, New Jersey, California, Texas, Virginia, and Georgia. The results of this survey showed that about 83% of Korean immigrants would go to Korea for cosmetic surgery, with 60% of them reporting their intention to visit Korea for dental care, back surgery, or infertility treatments. Later, another governmental report (KOTRA 2011) found that Korean immigrants, especially those with no have health insurance, often had a physical checkup when they visited Korea. They tended to have simple treatments or a cosmetic surgery rather than major surgeries in the home country. In addition to surveys, the Korean government also held exhibitions and conferences to attract Korean immigrant medical tourists. For example, in 2009, in order to promote the advantages of medical tours to Korea, the KIMA set up promotional booths at the Music Festival for Korean Immigrants in LA, one of the biggest festivals there.

The Korean government allows Korean immigrants who reside for a long enough time in the home country to apply for Korean national health insurance. When Korean immigrants plan to take medical tours, they can apply for Korean national health insurance using the following steps. First, they must submit a Domestic Residence Report form to the jurisdictional immigration office. About two weeks later, they will receive a domestic residence card. Three months after their admission to Korea, with their domestic residence card, Korean immigrants can apply for Korean national health insurance. Having Korean national health insurance would be one of contributing factors to Korean immigrants' medical tours to the home country because, with the national health insurance, they could receive medical care for much lower prices than they could get in the United States.

Korean local governments also made great efforts to attract more Korean immigrant medical tourists. Their main strategy was to make the MOUs with Korean associations in the United States so that these associations could send Korean immigrants to the hospitals in a sister city in Korea. Noticeably, Busan Metropolitan City signed the MOU with the Federation of Korean Associations, USA in 2009 (Park 2009b). Based on this MOU, Korean immigrants could receive a 10–50% discount on medical bills when they received medical care in Busan. In 2010, Daegu, the third largest city in Korea, held a business convention for *Hansang*, entrepreneurs from Korean diaspora communities, and hospitals in Daegu agreed on the MOU with many Korean immigrant associations. For instance, Daegu signed the MOU with the Federation of Korean Associations, USA, expecting many Korean immigrants to come to Daegu for medical care because Daegu had about 30% cheaper medical costs than Seoul.

## Private Sector Agencies

Korean hospitals and Korean travel agencies in the United States were two major private sector agencies who had various strategies to promote Korean immigrants' medical tourism. Much lower medical costs in Korea, a substantial proportion of uninsured Korean immigrants, and the lack of systematic check-up programs in the United States were the major important reasons for the Korean hospitals' targeting of Korean immigrants (Ahn and

Hurh 2009; Kim 2011). Several major Korean hospitals sent staff members to the US metropolitan areas with large Korean populations to publicize their superior medical services. In 2009, the Hanyang University Hospital staff members visited New York, Chicago, Los Angeles, San Francisco, and Seattle to publicize their medical tourism programs, which were designed for Korean immigrants (Choi 2010a). The Hanyang University Hospital also offered discounted flight tickets for Korean immigrants in these five areas in the United States so that they could save their expenses (Ahn and Hurh 2009). In addition, the Gangnam Severance Hospital offered fast-track services for Korean immigrants who had time pressure. Using fast-track services, Korean immigrants could avoid any waiting period for their examinations and treatments. They could also receive the results of their checkups quickly (Ahn and Hurh 2009).

In particular, some of the hospitals used a special strategy to attract more Korean immigrants to their hospitals: opening their branch offices in the United States. The Seoul National University (SNU) Hospital was the first one who opened a medical tourism office in the Korea Town of LA in 2008. Korean immigrants who were interested in receiving medical care at the SNU Hospital could consult with the dispatched nurses from Korea. There were 829 Korean immigrants who took medical tours through this LA office in 2009, and the number of them increased to over 1,000 in 2010 (Kim 2011). Additionally, the SNU Hospital established another branch office in Manhattan in 2012 to attract more Korean immigrants in the East Coast.

During the prosperity period (2009–2011) of medical tourism, other Korean hospitals also established branch offices in the LA area and the NY-NJ area where about 40% of Korean immigrants were concentrated in the United States. Following the SNU Hospital, the Catholic University of Korea Seoul St. Mary's Hospital opened a branch office in LA in 2010 and dispatched Dr. Jang, a plastic surgeon there. About 300 Korean immigrants, mostly from the LA area, took medical tours to this hospital in 2010. Their ability to consult with the medical doctor prior to their medical tourism is believed to have been the key factor to the success of the hospital in recruiting Korean immigrant clients. Another mega hospital, the Asan Medical Center, also opened branch offices in LA (2009) and New York (2010) to attract Korean immigrants who were interested in medical tourism to the home country.

Some hospitals stationed staff members at local travel agencies in the United States rather than established branch offices. For example, in 2010, the Asan Medical Center sent a staff member at Dongbu Tours in New York so that Korean immigrants who were interested in medical tourism could consult with a member of the hospital. In the following year, Yonsei Severance Hospital sent a nurse to Samho Tour in LA so that she could consult the Korean immigrants' health issues and build a special medical tourism program for them.

However, except for the first branch office of the SNU Hospital in the LA area, all other branch offices were shut down due to the low return on investment as of 2013. The demand for Korean immigrants' medical tourism has decreased naturally over time because some of them already had taken medical tours to the home country. Since they did not receive check-up services or major medical treatments frequently, the number of Korean immigrant medical tourists decreased as time passed. Also, they could have other routes to arrange their medical tourism than contacting hospitals. As will be examined in chapter 5, only about 4% of my survey respondents who participated in medical tourism reported that their medical tourism was arranged via hospital branch offices or the hospital websites.

Travel agencies in the United States were other private sector organizations who put a lot of efforts to promote Korean immigrants' medical tourism to the home country. In particular, two large travel agencies in United States (Aju and Samho Tour) conducted surveys on Korean immigrants' medical tourism to Korea. Their joint analysis showed that medical tourism packages successfully settled in the United States as one of the tour packages among Korean immigrants for both travel agencies (Choi 2010a). In 2009, Samho Tour sent 602 Korean immigrants to Yonsei Severance Hospital, and Aju Tour sent 143 Koreans to Asan Medical Center.

The big travel agencies, Aju, Samho, and Dongbu Tour, aggressively signed the MOU with Korean hospitals. Aju Tour, who introduced the medical tour packages for the first time to Korean immigrants in the United States, signed MOU with the Inha University Hospital (2007) and several other hospitals in Korea. Samho Tour, another travel agency based in the LA area, made an MOU with the Inha University Hospital (2007), Yonsei Severance Hospital (2009), Nune Eye Hospital (2011), and Serion Global Dermatologic and Aesthetic Surgery Center (2011). Lastly, Dongbu Tour, which was based in the NY-NJ area, agreed on the MOU with the Catholic University of Korea Yeouido St. Mary's Hospital (2009) and Asan Medical Center (2010).

In addition to these big tour agencies, other small travel agencies in the NY-NJ area did so and so. I interviewed ten employees who worked for these small travel agencies in NY-NJ area, asking them several questions about medical tourism. Most informants told me that they began to sell medical tourism packages since 2009 and that the number of Korean immigrant medical tourists reached its peak in 2011 and then declined rapidly. Thus, Korean immigrants' medical tours to Korea have gone through the same change as non-Korean foreign patients' medical tours to Korea.

Despite the decline in the number of Korean immigrants who bought medical tourism packages, many travel agency staff members told me that they still had special strategies to send more Korean immigrants to Korea for medical care. For example, one travel agency offered a customized program for each individual. A travel agency employee in his late 50s said:

> The price of the regular checkup is fixed (e.g., US$480 for women), but you can have an additional physical examination if you pay more. You can choose any examination or treatment if you want. You can choose an airline between the Korean Airline and the Asiana Airlines. You can choose any hospital from the list of 10,000 hospitals that are affiliated with this travel agency. From Yonsei Severance and Samsung Hospital to small doctor's office, you name it. If you choose Yonsei Severance Hospital, then I will contact the department of treatment for overseas and make an appointment for you. Then I will receive a confirmation email, and with that email, I can get a discount when I purchase a flight ticket for you. For example, it costs about US$1,500 from New York to Seoul if you fly with the Korean Airline, but if you choose a hospital which is affiliated with the Korean Airline, then the flight ticket will be US$1,300.

Except for the personalized services, advertising through local Korean newspapers was their only other strategy. A staff at a travel agency located on 32nd Street in Manhattan mentioned that usually four or five small travel agencies paid together for the advertisement in a local ethnic newspaper. Under the big advertisement section, each travel agency has its own address, phone number, and medical tourism packages.

## The Korean Community

The Korean community in the United States also supported Korean immigrants' medical tours to the home country. In particular, the Korean umbrella organizations in different areas in the United States played a significant role by signing MOUs with various Korean hospitals to give benefits to Korean immigrants. For example, the Korean American Association of Greater New York (KAAGNY) made an agreement with the Korea Association of Health Promotion (KAHP) in 2004, even before the revision of the medical law. Based on this agreement, the members of KAAGNY could receive a checkup for discounted prices at the KAHP. The year 2009 was a monumental year for medical tourism in Korea, as well as the Korean community in the NY-NJ area regarding Korean immigrants' medical tourism. The KAAGNY signed the MOU with three Korean hospitals in 2009. First, it established the MOU with Hallym University Medical Center, which offered Korean immigrants discounted medical bills and deferred payments for their medical care. Based on the MOU between the KAAGNY and Korea University Medical Center, the members of KAAGNY could receive discounted medical bills. The Wooridul Hospital, which signed the MOU with the KAAGNY, provided fast medical services, allowing Korean immigrants to test and see the results on the same day. Lastly, in 2011, the KAAGNY agreed on the MOU with the Kyung Hee University Medical Center so that their members could ask questions to doctors in Korea via Fax.

The Korean Produce Association (KPA) is another who contributed to Korean immigrants' medical tourism. In 2012, the KPA hosted the Korea Global Medical Tourism Expo at the Korean Harvest and Folklore Festivals for the first time (Kim 2012). About 50 Korean local governments, hospitals, and travel agencies participated in the expo to publicize their medical tourism programs to Korean immigrants and the non-Koreans who visited there.

## THE CONSEQUENCES OF MEDICAL TOURISM IN KOREA

With the Korean government's and private sector agencies' efforts to promote medical tourism, the number of foreign patients has soared since 2009, although their numbers were not collected by the Korean government until 2009. Prior to the revision of the medical laws, it was illegal to invite foreign patients to Korea. Based on the official government report (Statistics on International Patients in Korea, KHIDI 2016), the number of foreign patients who visited Korea for medical care was 60,201 in 2009. After the new medical laws went into effect, the number of foreign patients more than doubled (122,297) by 2011, more than tripled (211,218) by 2013, more than quadrupled (266,501) by 2014, and more than sextupled (364,189) by 2016.

Based on the 2016 KHIDI report, various countries have sent patients to Korea for medical care. In 2009, patients from 141 countries participated in medical tourism to Korea. The number of sending countries increased from 163 in 2010 to 187 in 2016. In 2016, China sent the most patients as it sent 127,648 patients, which is 35.2% of all foreign patients. The United States ranked the second in the number of patients sent to Korea. About 48,788 American patients came to receive medical care in Korea, comprising about 13.4% of all foreign patients in Korea in 2016. As indicated in Introduction, Korean immigrants who visit the home country as naturalized American citizens were not captured in the statistics of foreign patients. Most American patients were highly likely to be Korean immigrants with American citizenship (Jin 2011; Oh et al. 2014). In 2016, Japan and Russia each sent more than 25,000 patients to Korea, following China and the United States.

According to the Statistics on International Patients in Korea (KHIDI 2016), foreign patients received medical treatments often in the internal medicine departments (20.0%), plastic surgery department (11.3%), dermatology department (11.1%), check-up departments (9.3%), Ob/Gyn department (5.4%), and orthopedics (5.7%). About 4.2% of foreign patients received

*Hanbang* treatments, and 3.1% of them received dental treatments in Korea. The received medical treatments are different by patients' origin country. Noticeably, Chinese and Japanese patients showed a high prevalence of receiving esthetic-related treatments, such as plastic surgeries or skin treatments in Korea. For example, Japanese accounted for the significant proportion (44.0%) of those who had skin treatments, along with Chinese patients (13.5%). There was no governmental report that officially indicated reasons for foreign patients' medical tours to Korea. However, as examined earlier, the Korean government and private sector agencies tried to connect *Hallyu* to medical tourism to attract Japanese and Chinese patients who were interested in these elective care. Thus, it is assumed that Japanese and Chinese patients' high chance of receiving plastic surgeries or skin care in Korea were closely related to *Hallyu*.

Foreign patients have brought economic benefits as well as economic changes in Korea. The governmental report, Statistics on International Patients in Korea (KHIDI 2016), presents that the total medical profit generated by foreign patients has increased over time. Approximately US$103,200,000 was generated in 2010 and it more than doubled between 2010 and 2012 (US$267,300,000). Foreign patients generated about US$393,400,000 of medical profits for Korea in 2013, US$556,900,000 in 2014, US$669,400,000 in 2015, and finally US$860,600,000 in 2016. The average medical expenses per capita also increased over time too. On average, foreign patients spent about US$1,310 in 2010, but the amount increased to US$1,490 in 2011 and US$1,680 in 2012. In 2013, foreign patients spent about US$1,860 per capita, and they spent about 70% more than what Korean patients spent (KHIDI 2013). The amount of medical expenses that one foreign patient spent was over US$2,000 in 2014 and has increased to US$2,360 as of 2016.

The economic consequences of medical tourism were not just limited to Korea. They also brought various economic changes in several sending countries including the United States. For example, due to Korean immigrants' medical tour to the home country, some American health insurance companies changed their policies so that the US medical tourists, mostly Korean immigrants, can utilize their American insurance in Korea. For example, the Blue Cross Blue Shield of South Carolina announced to offer benefits for 10 surgeries performed at the Yonsei Severance Hospital in Seoul (Lee 2009). The UMR is the largest third-party administrator (TPA) for US companies and their Korean Association Preferred Health Plan provides claim administration for Korean-based companies with 25 or more employees in the United States. Individuals who belong to this program can access United Healthcare networks in the United States. Furthermore, they can be compensated for medical care in Korea. In addition, ILWI has launched a health plan that offers options with no deductible in the United States as well as medical tourism in Korea, with the goal of helping middle-aged Korean immigrants who are experiencing financial difficulties (Yoo 2010). In 2011, the Prime Medical Solutions, a medical tourism service company, introduced a new insurance program that included an option of medical tours to Korea (Chung 2011a).

Several new corporations have been formed as a result of medical tourism. For instance, Pacific Medline, a medical tourism agency in LA, was founded to send patients from Orange County to Korea (Moon 2009). In the NY-NJ area, several medical tourism consulting firms have appeared. The SK Management Consulting company built a portal website specializing in medical tourism, and Medical Fly Korea was established to connect American patients to Korean hospitals specializing in the treatment of cancer or spinal diseases (Choi 2010b).

In Korea, medical tourism has created new jobs, government-issued certificates, and college majors. A new occupation, the international medical tourism coordinator, has appeared in newspapers since 2007 and especially since 2009. Each year, Korean daily newspapers have published articles about this new job, explaining how to become medical tourism coordinators, how much they earn, and what kinds of work they do. Park (2009a) reported that medical tourism coordination has become of the most promising occupations. Since 2013, individuals who want to obtain a license to become an international medical tourism coordinator can take a national examination provided by Human Resources Development Service of Korea, which is an official governmental organization. This examination covers various subjects, including patient administration, medical tourism concepts, medical laws, and medical services.

In addition to the appearance of medical tourism coordinators, several schools have introduced new majors and programs related to medical tourism. For example, Masan University has established the Department of Medical Tourism and Chinese (Choi 2012). Students admitted to this department need to study the Chinese language as well as medical tourism in order to serve Chinese patients. Even a high school now offers courses in medical tourism: Joogmun High School on Jeju Island has courses in medical tourism, medical information, and health nursing (Oh 2010).

## PROBLEMS RELATED TO MEDICAL TOURISM

Some problems related to medical tourism have emerged with the growing popularity of medical tourism in Korea. These issues received the most attention from the government and the media during the stagnation period. In their articles, Hurh et al. (2013) and Kim, Lee, and Jung (2013) commonly pointed out problems and weaknesses of medical tourism in Korea, such as lack of legal systems, lack of professionals including medical tourism coordinators and translators, and uncentralized governmental agencies to support medical tourism. According to a staff member who is responsible for foreign patients at Asan Medical Center:

> Based on the feedback from our foreign patients from different countries, they are satisfied with our hospital's facilities, medical equipment, and the quality of doctors. However, they reveal concerns about communication and inpatient services. One of the biggest problems pointed out by them is that there are not many translators who can properly communicate with foreign patients and doctors, nurses, and staff members at the hospital.

A few newspaper articles reported on problems arising from medical tourism. The most frequently noted problems are the illegal brokers' exaggerated advertisements and high commissions (Bae 2012), and foreign patients being overcharged (Kim and Kang 2012). In particular, many Chinese patients have been charged more than Korean patients (Kim and Kang 2012). The excessive regulations against medical tourism, non-systematic connections between medical treatment and shopping/sightseeing, the scarcity of English road signs, and overcharge against foreign patients were reported as other problems of medical tourism in Korea.

In addition to foreign patients, Korean immigrants also faced problems during their medical tours to the home country. The most frequently noted problem was that Korean hospitals often forced Korean immigrants to receive unnecessary treatments or extra examinations (Ahn, Kim, and Hurh 2009; Kim and Ham 2012). Since Korean immigrants have been away from the home country for a while, they have become less familiar with Korean medical systems as well. Therefore, when Korean hospitals forced them to get unnecessary medical treatments, it was hard for them to resist. One Korean immigrant couple who participated in medical tourism showed their disappointment with medical tourism experiences because they paid extra US$6,000 for the additional examinations and treatments (Kim and Ham 2012).

Moreover, it was difficult to mediate any medical disputes between Korean immigrants and the hospitals because Korean immigrants did not usually stay in the home country for long periods of medical care. Due to the difficulty of arbitration of medical conflicts, Korean hospitals preferred to operate simple checkups to Korean immigrants rather than major surgeries which might cause serious medical disputes (Ahn, Kim, and Hurh 2009). Lastly, a few Korean immigrants were misdiagnosed with cancers during their medical tourism (Kim and Ham 2012). This was particularly important because the cancer screening was the most preferred healthcare that Korean immigrants wanted to receive during their medical tourism (Choi 2010c). As previously noticed, it was hard for Korean immigrants to ask for compensation for the misdiagnosis to the hospital because most of them did not stay in Korea for an extended period of time. Other kinds of problems Korean immigrants face during and after their medical tours to the home country will be discussed in chapter 5.

# *Chapter 3*

# Korean Immigrants' Healthcare Behaviors in the United States

## BARRIERS AND DIFFICULTIES TO FORMAL US HEALTHCARE

Before examining Korean immigrants' healthcare behaviors, including their medical tours to the home country, it is important to know the barriers to healthcare they encounter in the United States as they are assumed to be associated with the behaviors. As reviewed in chapter 1, previous studies have found that Korean immigrants face various structural, financial, and personal barriers to healthcare in the United States (Choi 2013; De Gagne et al. 2014; Jang, Kim, and Chiriboga 2005; Ryu, Young, and Park 2001; Shin 2002; Song et al. 2010). Confirming these earlier findings, more than half of the survey respondents answered that they had at least one barrier to formal US healthcare. Remarkably, 15% of all survey respondents who had received medical care in the United States reported that they encountered more than two barriers. The two most frequently cited combinations of the barrier were the language barrier and having no insurance, followed by the language barrier and cultural differences.

Table 3.1 shows that language barrier was the most common barrier for Korean immigrants in obtaining healthcare in the United States. Since more than half of the survey respondents said they spoke very little or no English, it is not surprising that more than one-third of the survey respondents reported that they experienced a language barrier when they received medical care in the United States. In addition to the language barrier, survey respondents pointed out other barriers, such as uninsured status, cultural differences, and perceived racial discrimination. A few survey respondents indicated additional obstacles, such as having difficulty in making appointments, long wait times, complicated referral processes, and poor medical equipment at doctors' offices.

**Table 3.1 Types of Korean Immigrants' Barriers and Difficulties to Healthcare in the United States**

| *Barriers or Difficulties* | N | % |
|---|---|---|
| None | 205 | 44.5 |
| Language barriers | 158 | 34.3 |
| Having no insurance | 113 | 24.5 |
| Cultural differences | 45 | 9.8 |
| Other barriers | 25 | 5.5 |
| Total[1] | 546 | 118.6 |

[1]The respondents who have never received medical care in the US are excluded in this analysis ($N$ = 461). Since several respondents ($N$ = 73) gave multiple answers, the sum of the responses exceeds 100%.
*Source*: Survey of 507 Korean immigrants in the NY-NJ area.

Analysis of the in-depth interviews revealed four types of language barriers in healthcare: (1) difficulties in understanding medical terminology in English, (2) difficulties in describing their symptoms in English, (3) difficulties in communicating with non-Korean doctors, and (4) feeling powerless in their interactions with non-Korean doctors. First two types will be discussed in this section because they have more *linguistic* aspects, whereas last two types emphasize more *interpersonal* aspects. Last two types will be discussed in the next section when I examine Korean immigrants' preference for co-ethnic doctors as their preference is related to the doctor-patient relationship.

First, some interviewees reported that it was hard for them to understand difficult medical terminology in English. They were anxious about their inability to understand English medical terminology at hospitals, and their anxiety often led them to choose co-ethnic doctors. Second, for some Korean immigrants, the ability to describe their symptoms in English was limited. In their view, due to their limited English, they did not know enough English adjectives or other words to accurately describe their pain. For example, Min-Seok Kim, a middle-aged employee at a Korean community center, explained that he knew various adjectives to describe pain in Korean. Additionally, many Korean-language phrases or words used to describe certain kinds of pain or other symptoms simply do not have direct English translations. However, since he knew only one word—pain—to describe his discomfort in English, it was hard for him to elaborate on his pain to American doctors. Since Korean doctors understood his expressions or descriptions right away, he preferred to see Korean doctors or return to Korea for medical care.

When I asked to identify any difficulties or barriers, another informant, who has lived in the United States for 40 years, reported a similar problem:

> I am confident in understanding and speaking English in my everyday life. But, elaborating symptoms in English is delicate and challenging. For example, regarding a stomachache, I may have a slight pain, a plucking-off pain, or other kinds of pain. However, I can only say "it hurts" in English. A headache is the

same. I can say "I have a headache, or I have pain in my head," but that was it. I cannot describe it in any detail. (Young-Sik Chung, 67, business owner, Fort Lee, New Jersey)

The second most popular barrier was having no health insurance in the United States. About a quarter of survey respondents answered that their uninsured status was a major obstacle to their healthcare utilization. Since they had lived in Korea, which offers very affordable national health insurance for all people, many of them revealed their hesitance to pay for more expensive health insurance in the United States. For example, a 40-year-old nonsmoker who earns US$30,000 a year will pay about US$4,500 a year (US$372 per month for 12 months = US$4,464) for the second lowest cost plan in New York state (Cox et al. 2015). By contrast, an employee in Korea who earns about US$30,000 pays only about US$1,800 annually for his/her health insurance, as Korean national health insurance contribution rate is only about 6% of his/her salary (Song 2009). Korean immigrants' having to pay large out-of-pocket amounts for medical care due to lack of health insurance along with other barriers have contributed to their major coping strategies which will be discussed in the later section.

About one-tenth of survey respondents reported that cultural differences made them feel uncomfortable when they received medical care in the United States. For example, Young-Ja Park, an elderly informant who immigrated two years ago, described how cultural differences made her feel scared at the hospital during the Halloween season:

My family doctor was a first-generation Korean, but I still had to see a non-Korean doctor to take an X-ray and MRI. Immediately after stepping into the American hospital, I became so scared. It was around the Halloween season, and the hospital's decoration was very scary. At the lobby, there was a statue overloaded with fake blood. Fake blood was everywhere at the hospital. When I saw it, I was freaked out. How could they do that at the hospital, especially in the country of Protestantism? The hospital decoration should make patients feel comfortable. (Young-Ja Park, 72, retired, Fort Lee, New Jersey)

Notably, some Korean women pointed out that they felt culturally different and that made them uncomfortable especially when they had Ob/Gyn examinations in the United States. Seong-Sook Kim, a 45-year-old woman who had been in the United States for about ten years, recounted her first experience at Ob/Gyn. When the doctor asked her, "When did you have sex for the first time?" she had a cultural shock and felt very uncomfortable telling him about her past sexual experiences. Another female informant in her late 30s also felt embarrassed and upset at the Ob/Gyn:

When I had an abnormal period cycle after arriving in the US, I went to the Ob/Gyn. The American doctor had several tests on me. He had an internal examination on my virginal, and it hurt badly. I could not understand why he did an internal examination because I told him that I had no sexual experience before. In Korea, doctors did not take an internal examination of a virgin because they were afraid of causing her to lose hymen. I think Americans undervalue the loss of hymen than Koreans. I felt very upset for losing it unexpectedly. (Ji-Young Kim, 39, employee at a Korean firm, Flushing, Queens)

Only a few respondents (2.2%) noted that their perceived racial discrimination made them difficult in utilizing healthcare in the United States. Some Korean immigrants reported their perceived discrimination especially by non-Korean receptionists at the front desk. For example, a 32-year-old female respondent described her experience of racial discrimination at the hospital. She argued that she encountered racial discrimination not from white American doctors, but from the non-white staff members who worked at the counter when she did check-in or check-out processes. Another informant even changed her family doctor because of the attitude of the Latino and Black staff members at the physician's office:

> I changed my family doctor and my Ob/Gyn doctor not because of the doctor but because of the attitude of receptionists. They were very unkind and browbeaten me when I did not understand what they were saying. It might sound racist, but the horrible receptionists were all Latino and Black. I have never felt that the doctor disregarded me, but they (receptionists) did. That was the reason for me to change the doctor. They discriminated against me not only for my imperfect language but also because of my Asian background. (Tae-Sook Lee, 38, housewife, Bronx, New York)

As shown, more than half of Korean immigrants suffer from various obstacles in utilizing healthcare in the United States. Language barriers, lack of health insurance, and other barriers have contributed to their major coping strategies: (1) seeing co-ethnic doctors for better communication and discounted medical bills; (2) practicing *Hanbang*, as it is relatively cheaper than Western medicine, although not covered by insurance; and (3) medical tours to Korea for various reasons, such as cheaper medical care, easier communication, and more comfortable feeling in the home country.

## PREFERENCE FOR CO-ETHNIC DOCTORS AND DEPENDENCY ON THEM

As mentioned in chapter 1, immigrants generally prefer and seek co-ethnic physicians due to their shared language and culture and the immigrants' limited knowledge of Western medicine. Korean immigrant respondents also expressed their great preference for co-ethnic doctors in the United States. Based on the number of medical offices that appeared in the Korea Daily Business Directory (2014), there are 1,124 Korean medical offices open in the NY-NJ area, which include Western-style medical offices and dental offices that fall within formal healthcare system, as well as informal healthcare offices, such as *Hanbang* and chiropractic offices. Of these, 488 were Western-style medical offices, comprising nearly half (43.4%) of all Korean medical offices in the NY-NJ area; 322 dental offices make up 28.7% of all Korean medical offices, whereas 196 *Hanbang* offices account for 17.4%. Chiropractic offices ($N$ = 118) account for about 10.5% of NY-NJ Korean medical offices. Considering that about 250,000 Koreans live in the NY-NJ area, roughly one Korean medical office in this area is available for every 200 Koreans. These figures may explain Korean immigrants' great preference for co-ethnic doctors and their heavy dependence on them.

The analysis of survey and interview data also supported earlier findings that indicated Korean immigrants' preference for co-ethnic doctors (Choi 2013; De Gagne et al. 2014; Son 2013). About two-thirds (64.5%) of all survey respondents preferred Korean doctors, whereas only 5% of them preferred non-Korean doctors. About a quarter of them showed no preference regarding the physician's ethnicity, and 6% of them answered that their preference depends on the type of medical care. In most cases, they preferred Korean doctors for dental care because they believed that Korean dentists were more dexterous than American dentists. As will be indicated in chapter 5, their preference for Korean dentists was closely related to the fact that dental care was the second most popular medical treatments that Korean immigrants received in Korea.

In a previous study, Portes and his associates (2012) mentioned that when immigrants have limited English proficiency or have cultural differences as barriers, they would be likely to see co-ethnic doctors as coping strategies. Other studies (Choi 2013; De Gagne et al. 2014; Son 2013) pointed out that Korean immigrants prefer Korean doctors mostly due to their language barriers. As shown earlier, Table 3.1 shows that the language barrier was the biggest obstacle for Korean immigrants to get medical care in the United States, and it strongly affected their inclination to choose Korean doctors. In the first section of this chapter, I discussed two types of language barriers that are more linguistic in nature, such as difficulties in understanding medical terminology in English and expressing symptoms in English. In this section, I examine the other two types of language barriers that are more interpersonal and related to their preference for co-ethnic doctors.

Some Korean informants noted that communicating with non-Korean doctors in English was often confusing because it was difficult for them to catch the nuance in a doctor's words. When the doctor said "you will be all right" after a medical test, it was often hard for Korean patients to judge whether the physician said this because he believed the test results to be fine or he just wanted to reassure them about expected bad results. Moreover, difficulties in communication exposed Korean immigrants to challenging situations at the hospital. For example, Ji-Hoon, a male interviewee in his late 40s, explained that it was hard for him to argue with healthcare professionals because of the difficulty in conversing with them:

> A few years ago, I fractured my rib when I went skiing. The person who took the X-ray was a white man at the emergency room. Even after several hours, he and other staff members could not find the fracture after taking thousands of X-rays of me. I was very upset at them because of their incompetence. However, I could not argue with them because I had difficulty in communicating with them. My English proficiency was not good enough to make them apologize to me, which I thought was a divine right of a patient. After that experience, I have always tried to find a Korean doctor. My doctors have to be Korean. (Ji-Hoon Park, 45, college staff member, Flushing, Queens)

Lastly, some informants indicated that there were power issues when their doctors were not Korean. Bo-Hee Kim, a 37-year-old woman who had lived in the United States for ten years, said that she felt inferior to the American doctors when she spoke to them in English. Usually, doctors have more power than their patients because they have better medical knowledge, and she indicated that the power imbalance was even more severe between her and non-Korean speaking doctors because of the language barrier. By contrast, when she spoke in Korean to Korean doctors, she felt that she had almost the same level of power. Another female informant reported that the power imbalance between an immigrant patient and a non-co-ethnic physician became worse when a patient was younger and female. From her experiences with non-Korean doctors, age, and gender, in addition to language barriers, contributed to her feeling powerless in front of native English-speaking male doctors:

> When I saw a Korean doctor, I felt that we were equal. I could elaborate all of my symptoms in detail. However, when I saw an American physician, I felt that I was inferior to him. Moreover, since I am a female patient and younger than almost all American doctors, I felt they looked down on me. (Ji-Min Lee, 34, artist, Manhattan, New York)

In addition to language barriers, having no health insurance was another reason for their preference for Korean doctors. As indicated earlier, about one-third of survey respondents were not insured in the United States. For these uninsured Korean immigrants, getting a discounted medical bill by paying cash was a primary reason for looking for Korean doctors. They also felt more comfortable discussing their uninsured status with Korean doctors.

A female interviewee in her late 50s mentioned that she had seen Korean doctors for more than 20 years because she has never had health insurance in the United States. She said that Korean doctors, as immigrants themselves, understood her uninsured situation better than native-born American doctors. Dong-Joo, an elderly man who did not have health insurance in the United States, emphasized that paying a medical bill in cash was a win-win strategy for both Korean patients and Korean doctors:

> The language barrier was the first reason for my search for a Korean doctor. The second reason was medical costs. When I went to see a Korean doctor, I could get a discounted medical bill if I paid it in cash. It was mutual help between a patient and a doctor because he could also have some financial benefits if patients paid the bill in cash. It was a tacit promise between Korean patients and doctors, and it was what I did with my Korean doctor. (Dong-Joo Han, 67, retired, Fort Lee, New Jersey)

Researchers (Wang 2007; Wang, Rosenberg, and Lo 2008) have found a discrepancy between Chinese immigrants' preference for Chinese-speaking doctors and their actual prevalence of seeing them because of the geographical distance between where Chinese immigrants lived (suburbs) and the location of Chinese doctors (downtown). Unlike Chinese immigrants, Korean immigrants in the NY-NJ area showed consistency between their preference for co-ethnic doctors and their actual visits to co-ethnic doctors probably due to the large numbers of Korean doctors in the area as indicated earlier. Except for the 35% of survey respondents who did not have a family doctor, the vast majority of Korean immigrants had co-ethnic doctors as their family doctors regardless of whether the Korean doctors were immigrants or not. Nearly half (46.3%) had first-generation Korean doctors, and about 40% had 1.5- or second-generation Korean doctors as their family physicians. By contrast, only 14% had non-Koreans as their family doctors.

More informants preferred first-generation Korean immigrant doctors to younger-generation Korean doctors, but they still felt more comfortable with 1.5- or second-generation Korean doctors than with non-Korean doctors, even if they communicated with the younger-generation Korean doctors in English, because of similarities in culture:

> My family doctor was a second-generation Korean American, and he did not speak Korean very well. However, I still felt more relaxed with him than with American doctors. We communicated 85% in English and 15% in Korean. When I had to explain my symptom in English, I often spoke in Korean to him, and he understood it most of the time. Of course, he, as a second-generation Korean American, did not fully understand my Korean. However, his understanding of Korean culture helped our communication in Korean. (Mi-Jin Noh, 34, florist, Flushing, Queens)

## PRACTICE OF *HANBANG*

As previously noted in chapter 1, health researchers suggested that CAM, which is also called as traditional medicine, oriental medicine, folk medicine, or *Hanbang*, is one of the healthcare options for Asian immigrants. In the previous section, I indicated that there were about 200 *Hanbang* offices in the NY-NJ area which comprise about 17% of all medical offices. When the number of *Hanbang* offices was divided by the number of Korean immigrants in this area, there are about one *Hanbang* offices per 1,100 Korean immigrants. About 15% of all survey respondents practiced *Hanbang* in the United States in last five years. This percent was reasonable when the proportion of *Hanbang* offices (17%) among all medical offices in the NY-NJ area was taken into account. Moreover, the proportion of my survey respondents who practiced *Hanbang* was similar to that reported by Kim and Chan (2004). In their study, about 15% of Korean immigrants preferred *Hanbang* to Western medicine.

The analysis of my survey data is similar to what previous scholars (Chin 1992; Han 2001; Kim et al. 2002; Pourat et al. 1999) have found: middle-aged and elderly Korean immigrants were more likely to practice *Hanbang* than younger Koreans. As Table 3.2 shows, older Korean immigrants showed a greater tendency to receive *Hanbang* treatments than younger Korean immigrants. In particular, middle-aged Korean immigrants who were 50 to 64 years old showed the highest percent of practicing *Hanbang* than all other age groups. In addition to them, those who were in their 40s or those who were elderly also showed a great tendency of utilizing *Hanbang* than their younger counterparts.

I suspect that there are several reasons for older Koreans' greater propensity of practicing *Hanbang*. Most of all, they are more likely to be ill due to their older age, so they are more likely to receive any treatments, including *Hanbang* treatments. Also, *Hanbang* treatments are closely related to geriatric illnesses (e.g., back pain, knee pain, and arthritis). Lastly, as will be discussed later, middle-aged Korean immigrants had the greatest prevalence of practicing *Hanbang* due to their uninsured status. If they were retired before reaching the age of 65, they were not eligible to receive Medicare. Since *Hanbang* treatment is not covered by health insurance in the United States, they may choose *Hanbang* as one of the options for their healthcare.

The proportion of Korean immigrants who utilized *Hanbang* is lower compared to those who received any Western medical care in the Unites States in the last five years (77%). Nevertheless, a significant proportion of Korean immigrants has utilized *Hanbang* in the United States. According to my in-depth interviews, there are two main reasons for Korean immigrants' preference for and practice of *Hanbang*. First, some Korean immigrants

**Table 3.2 Practice of *Hanbang* by Age Group**

| | *Age Group* | | | | | |
|---|---|---|---|---|---|---|
| *Practice of Hanbang* | *18–29* | *30–39* | *40–49* | *50–64* | *65 Years Old or Older* | *Total* |
| No | 86 (95.6%) | 81 (83.5%) | 96 (82.1%) | 95 (81.2%) | 73 (84.9%) | 431 (85.0%) |
| Yes | 4 (4.4%) | 16 (16.5%) | 21 (17.9%) | 22 (18.8%) | 13 (15.1%) | 76 (15.0%) |
| Total | 90 (100.0%) | 97 (100.0%) | 117 (100.0%) | 117 (100.0%) | 86 (100.0%) | 507 (100.0%) |

$\chi^2$ (4, $N$ = 507) = 10.17, $p$ = < .05/ gamma = .18.
*Source*: Survey of 507 Korean immigrants in the NY-NJ area.

prefer *Hanbang* treatments because they believe that it understands the fundamental constitution of their body better than Western medicine. In their view, *Hanbang* is a more suitable therapy to cure their illness because it tries to fix the root cause of their illness by changing the physical constitution. For them, the Western medicine is just a temporary remedy as it reduces pain temporarily by using painkillers. By contrast, they believe that *Hanbang* suggests more preventive ways to patients to treat their illness. Hani Kim, a 30-year-old computer designer, asserted, "I trust *Hanbang* because it understands my constitution. If I go to see a Western doctor, he will give me the same medication that he gives to other people. However, if I go to see a doctor who practices *Hanbang*, he will give me a special treatment effective just for me." Young-Soo Kim, a college professor, emphasized the preventive aspect of *Hanbang* treatments:

> I prefer *Hanbang* to the western medicine because it is more preventive than western medicine. *Hanbang* changes the constitution of your body, whereas western medicine just restrains the pain of the disease by medicine. Since I had suffered from acid reflux for a while, I went to see a Korean doctor who practices Western medicine. For five years, he just gave me medicine that suppressed my acid reflux. After five years of western treatments, my reflux still had not been cured. So I went to see the *Hanui,* a doctor who practices *Hanbang*. He was surprised by the list of the medications that I took for last five years. Rather than taking medications, My *Hanui* suggested a special diet for me. He helped me to change my constitution in a more preventive way. After having *Hanbang* practices, my reflux had been much eased. (Young-Soo Kim, 70, college professor, Flushing, Queens)

Second, as expected, more Korean immigrants who indicated that they had encountered barriers to the US healthcare system used *Hanbang* in comparison to those who did not encounter any barriers. About 18% of those who encountered barriers practiced *Hanbang*, while about 11% of those who had no barriers practiced it. As Portes, Fernández-Kelly, and Light (2012) pointed out, my informants, especially those who did not have US health insurance, sought *Hanbang* for financial reasons. As noted in the previous section, about a quarter of survey respondents were found to have no health insurance in the United States. Since *Hanui* (*Hanbang* doctors) charge substantially lower fees than Western medical doctors, Korean immigrants with no insurance would rather visit *Hanbang* offices than Western medical offices. In particular, middle-aged Korean immigrants who were uninsured but not yet qualified for Medicare actively sought *Hanbang*. For example, Jae-Young Paek, a middle-aged woman who worked as a dental technician, explained that she saw *Hanui* for pain in her knee. She paid about US$50 per visit because her insurance did not cover *Hanbang* practice. However, she did not think the visits were too expensive because she would have paid about the same amount in co-pay if she had visited an orthopedic specialist. Hee-Jin Lee, a 38-year-old employee at a nonprofit organization, first sought an orthopedic doctor for acute pain in her back. However, the fees for consulting the doctor and getting an X-ray were about US$200. Alternatively, she called *Hanbang* offices listed in the Korean business directory and found the office that offered the lowest price, US$50 per treatment.

## MEDICAL TOURS TO THE HOME COUNTRY

The last coping strategy to offset barriers to formal US healthcare is to return to the home country for medical care. About a quarter (23.9%) of all survey respondents has ever visited Korea for medical care since their migration to the United States. Among Korean immigrants who participated in medical tourism, nearly half of them (51/121*100 = 42.1%) engaged in medical tourism just once. About one-third (45/121*100 = 37.2%) took medical tours two or three times, and about one-fifth (25/121*100 = 20.7%) had visited Korea four times or more frequently to receive medical treatments. There were four people who took ten or more medical tours to the home country, and all of them led very active and extreme transnational lives. For example, Hyun-Seok Choi, a middle-aged man who runs a fashion jewelry store in Manhattan, had the most frequent numbers of medical tourism visits among all informants. For business purposes, he has to visit Korea at least twice a year. Thus, since migrating to the United States in the 1990s, he has visited Korea more than 40 times. Since he had to take business trips frequently and regularly, he applied for Korean national health insurance and tried to get as many as medical treatments as possible while staying there. In other words, although he is a US citizen and spends most of his time in the United States, Korea has been the primary place for his medical care.

In chapter 2, I investigated the Korean government's and other private sectors' efforts to attract overseas Koreans to the home country for medical care. As pointed out, 2009 was a turning point year for medical tourism in Korea because the Korean government revised the medical law that made introducing, arranging, and inviting foreign patients legally. It seems that the revised medical law and Korean government's efforts positively influenced Korean immigrants' medical tours to the home country, although they cannot be directly measured; only 16 of 121 Korean immigrants who participated in medical tours (13.2%) took medical tours before 2009. Rather, the vast majority of them made medical tours in 2009 and after. More than half (54.5%) visited Korea in 2012 or later.

Conversations with my informants revealed that Korean immigrants' decisions to engage in medical tourism were highly or moderately associated with some of their barriers to US medical care and the first two healthcare behaviors that have been examined earlier. First, as expected, there was a significant association between having obstacles to US healthcare and taking medical tours to the home country. Table 3.3 shows that 84% of Korean immigrants with no barrier to US healthcare had never taken a medical tour to the homeland, while 71% of those with some barriers had never visited Korea for medical care. The difference between the two groups is more salient among people who took more frequent medical tours. About 17% of Korean immigrants who indicated any difficulty in accessing US healthcare had two or more medical tours to the home country; meanwhile, less than 10% of those who had no difficulties had taken two or more medical tours. This clearly shows that those who experienced difficulties utilizing US healthcare were more likely to engage in medical tourism as a coping mechanism.

Second, as expected, there was a positive association between preference for co-ethnic doctors and taking medical tours to the home country. As Table 3.4 shows, 18% of the Korean immigrants who did not prefer Korean doctors in the United States took at least one medical tour to the home country, compared to 27% of Korean immigrants who preferred Korean doctors. However, having a Korean family doctor in the United States was not significantly associated with the medical tourism experience. In fact, Korean immigrants who had co-ethnic family doctors had a lower rate of taking medical tours to the home country than those who had non-Korean family doctors. This finding suggests that Korean immigrants who could easily find co-ethnic doctors in their neighborhood in the NY-NJ area, which have many Korean doctors, did not need to go back to Korea to seek medical care since they could communicate effectively with their doctor in the same language, or at the very least, they shared culture.

**Table 3.3 Number of Medical Tours by Barriers to the Healthcare in the United States**

| *Number of Medical Tours* | *Having Any Barriers* | | |
|---|---|---|---|
| | *No Barrier* | *Any Barriers* | *Total* |
| None | 172 (83.5%) | 214 (71.1%) | 386 (76.1%) |
| Once | 15 (7.3%) | 36 (12.0%) | 51 (10.1%) |
| Twice or more | 19 (9.2%) | 51 (16.9%) | 70 (13.8%) |
| Total | 206 (100.0%) | 301 (100.0%) | 507 (100.0%) |

$\chi^2$ (2, $N$ = 507) = 10.41, $p$ = < .005/ gamma = .32.
*Source*: Survey of 507 Korean immigrants in the NY-NJ area.

**Table 3.4 Number of Medical Tours by Preference for Co-ethnic Doctors**

| *Number of Medical Tours* | *Preference for Korean Doctors* | | |
|---|---|---|---|
| | *No* | *Yes* | *Total* |
| None | 147 (81.7%) | 239 (73.1%) | 386 (76.1%) |
| Once | 18 (10.0%) | 33 (10.1%) | 51 (10.1%) |
| Twice or more | 15 (8.3%) | 55 (16.8%) | 70 (13.8%) |
| Total | 180 (100.0%) | 327 (100.0%) | 507 (100.0%) |

$\chi^2$ (2, $N$ = 507) = 7.17, $p < .05$/ gamma = .24.
*Source*: Survey of 507 Korean immigrants in the NY-NJ area.

Lastly, Korean immigrants who utilized *Hanbang* in the United States had a higher rate of taking medical tours to the home country than those who did not. Table 3.5 shows that about one-fifth of those who did not use *Hanbang* took at least one medical tour to Korea, compared to about one-third of who used *Hanbang*. This finding is consistent with Xing's (1998) argument that overseas Chinese' trust in traditional Chinese medicine contributed to overseas Chinese' medical tours to the home country. Like overseas Chinese, some Korean interviewees expressed their belief in the effectiveness of *Hanbang*, and that was often their primary reason for taking medical tours to the home country.

Interestingly, a few Korean informants reported that they preferred to receive *Hanbang* treatments in Korea rather than in the United States, although they still practiced it here. For them, distrust of academic credentials in the United States was the primary reason for their skepticism or reluctance. They argued that there were only a few universities in Korea, such as Kyung Hee University, which have *Hanbang* departments. It takes six years to complete a B.A. degree in *Hanbang*. Moreover, since it is very competitive to get admission to a school and become a *Hanui*, a doctor who gives *Hanbang* treatment, they are highly selective in Korea. By contrast, in their view, it is much easier to become a *Hanui* in the United States because there are more universities and two-year colleges which have Oriental medicine or Acupuncture departments. Also, they indicated that it takes a much shorter period of time to complete the degree in the United States. All of these reasons indicate that the respondents felt that standards were much lower for *Hanui* in the United States. Most of the Korean informants were aware of these differences, so they preferred to get *Hanbang* care in Korea rather than in the United States.

Yong-Gyu Lim, a middle-aged taxi driver, asserted that he visited Korea to receive *Chunwha* therapy, a particular type of *Hanbang* treatment because he believed that *Hanui* in Korea had more reliable academic credentials than *Hanui* in the United States:

> A few years ago, I had severe back pain. I even had health insurance in the US, but I still went back to Korea for treatments. I wanted to receive *Hanbang*

**Table 3.5 Number of Medical Tours by Practice of *Hanbang* in the United States**

| *Number of Medical Tours* | *Practicing* Hanbang *in the United States* | | |
|---|---|---|---|
| | *No* | *Yes* | *Total* |
| None | 337 (78.2%) | 49 (64.5%) | 386 (76.1%) |
| Once | 37 (8.6%) | 14 (18.4%) | 51 (10.1%) |
| Twice or more | 57 (13.2%) | 13 (17.1%) | 70 (13.8%) |
| Total | 431 (100.0%) | 76 (100.0%) | 507 (100.0%) |

$\chi^2$ (2, $N$ = 507) = 8.51, $p < .05$/ gamma = .27.
*Source*: Survey of 507 Korean immigrants in the NY-NJ area.

> treatments because I believed that *Hanbang* was better than western medicine. Then, I thought that *Hanui* in Korea had better ability than *Hanui* in the US because the majority of them graduated from a competitive university such as Kyung Hee University. By contrast, it was much easier to be *Hanui* in the US. If you spent two years at a community college somewhere in Long Island, you can get a license to be a *Hanui* in the US. That was the reason why I did not trust them as much as I trusted *Hanui* in Korea. (Yong-Gyu Lim, 58, taxi driver, Bayside, Queens)

In order to assess the reasons for medical tourism besides the barriers to formal US healthcare and other healthcare behaviors, I directly asked the following question to 121 survey respondents who have participated in medical tourism what factors contributed to their visit to Korea for the medical purpose. As Table 3.6 shows, about half of the respondents ($N$ = 62) gave two or more answers, suggesting that multiple reasons simultaneously affected their decision on medical tourism, rather than a single reason. For example, a 64-year-old female informant described the style of her medical tour as "the trinity style," because she chose Korea for faster, more accurate, and kinder medical care. Another middle-aged female interviewee, who migrated to the United States 20 years ago and who had US health insurance, also pointed out three reasons for her medical tourism: cheaper medical costs, less complicated system, and easier communications with healthcare professionals.

The most frequent single reason was lower medical costs in Korea. About 60% of the respondents reported that the relatively cheaper medical expenses contributed to their decision on medical tours to the home country. Personal interviews also support findings of the survey. For example, several informants had the same medical treatments in the United States and Korea. When they compared the costs of the same treatments in both countries, the medical expenses were much cheaper in Korea than the United States. Yeon-Joo Chung, a female informant in her mid-30s, had the same Ob/Gyn surgeries in both countries. For the same treatment, she spent about one thousand dollars more in the United States than in Korea, although she did not have a health insurance in either country. Sun-Hee Choi was another informant who was

**Table 3.6 Reasons for Medical Tourism**

| *Reasons* | *N* | % |
|---|---|---|
| Cheaper medical costs in Korea | 72 | 59.5 |
| Easier communications | 43 | 35.5 |
| Feel more comfortable in Korea | 39 | 32.2 |
| Simpler procedures in Korea | 34 | 28.1 |
| Better ability of doctors in Korea | 28 | 23.1 |
| A shorter waiting period | 24 | 19.8 |
| No health insurance in the United States | 22 | 18.2 |
| Other reasons | 27 | 22.3 |
| Total[1] | 289 | 238.7 |

[1]Since several respondents ($N = 62$) gave multiple answers, the sum of the answers exceeds 100%.
*Source*: Survey of 121 Korean immigrants who have participated in medical tourism to Korea.

surprised by the expensive medical costs in the United States for the same medical procedures:

> I have a US health insurance through my son's job. Nevertheless, I still went back to Korea for medical care due to expensive medical costs in the US. One day, I fell on the ice and I needed to take an X-ray here. The hospital claimed 4,000 dollars for an X-ray even though my son pays 500 dollars every month for my insurance! I was so surprised by how expensive it was. Because of expensive medical costs, I did not receive further treatments here. Instead, I took an X-ray again in Korea and received treatments there last year. In Korea, the whole medical procedures for the same medical issue cost only about few hundred dollars, even without a Korean national health insurance. (Sun-Hee Choi, 69, housewife, Palisades Park, New Jersey)

The second popular reason was easier communication with healthcare professionals; about one-third of respondents chose this reason. As pointed out earlier in this chapter, about one-third of Korean immigrants had language barriers in accessing the US healthcare system, and they were likely to choose this reason for medical tours to the home country. Another one-third of respondents replied that feeling more comfortable in Korea was the reason for their medical tourism. For them, receiving medical care was not just about the actual practice, but also something emotional. They, especially those who lived alone in the United States, felt comfortable getting medical care in the home country because their relatives and friends gave them emotional support. Kyung-Eun Park, a 56-year-old employee at a nonprofit organization in Flushing, said that she became weak-minded and homesick when she was ill. She said that her going back to the homeland for medical care was "like a bird who tries to be nestling in mother bird's arms." Not only emotional attachment but also Korea as a homogenous society made Korean immigrants more comfortable in the homeland. Sung-Joon Suh, a middle-aged employee at a Korean firm who took medical tours once in two years, commented, "Unlike in the US, I was not a minority member in Korea. In Korea, a homogenous society, I just looked like one of them. I was not physically distinctive in Korea as I was in the US. The fact that I looked just like everybody else made me feel so comfortable when I stayed in Korea for medical care."

Simpler medical procedures and a shorter waiting period in Korea were also important reasons for Korean immigrants' medical tourism. More than a quarter of Korean immigrant medical tourists (28%) recognized that medical procedures in the United States were more complicated than that in Korea. Since the Korean national health insurance offers the same coverage for all people despite the different insurance rates, they did not need to call the insurance company or the hospital to check if the hospital accepts their national health insurance. By contrast, it felt cumbersome to call American doctor's office before a visit to check if their insurance would be acceptable. To them, the check-in and the check-out processes were much easier in Korea because the hospital handled everything right after receiving patient's name and social security number.

Some informants also felt it was very inconvenient to visit different hospitals or doctors' offices for examination in the United States, whereas a checkup for the entire body in one hospital was possible in Korea. A 66-year-old male informant, who had been in the United States for 35 years and had five medical tours to Korea, complained that it took him several days to get examinations at different doctor's offices in the United States. By contrast, he spent only three hours for a whole checkup in Korea. Another elderly interviewee told me that he was amazed by the simple and fast the medical procedures in Korea:

> The main reason for my medical tours to Korea was convenience. I had a health insurance in the US, but medical procedures were too complicated here. I had to make an appointment with each department for a checkup. And I had to make separate visits to different doctors' offices for an endoscopy or an x-ray. That was very cumbersome. When I had a checkup at Inha University Hospital in Korea, I did not stay at the hospital even a day. I checked in at 8am and was discharged at 11am, after examining my whole body in one building. (Dae-Sik. Choi, 70, retired, Fort Lee, New Jersey)

Along with a simpler procedure, a shorter waiting period in Korea was another attractive factor to Korean immigrants' medical tourism. One-fifth of medical tourists reported that they decided to go back to Korea for medical care for a shorter waiting period. Joo-Hyun Lee, who had immigrated to the United States 20 years ago, took medical tours to the home country for a checkup and other medical care because it took a long time to get treatments and receive the results in the United States. She had to wait several weeks to see a doctor for a physical examination, waited another week to see the results and waited another week to get treated. She said, "Since I was quick in temper, I could not bear a long waiting period in American hospitals. I screamed at the receptionists and myself, 'quickly, quickly'!" She even said that she would go back to Korea if she found any severe disease because of a short waiting time, although she had a US insurance. Another informant said that a shorter waiting period was a strong pull factor to her medical tourism. She compared how long it took for her to make an appointment, get treatment, and see the results for the same disease in the United States and Korea:

> I had a same Ob/Gyn examination both in the US and Korea. It took several weeks for me to see a doctor to get examined in the US. By contrast, doctors in Korea were more flexible, so I was able to see a doctor right after calling them. Also, it took several months for me to see the results in the US, whereas it took only 30 minutes in Korea. (Ji-Won Cha, 36, accountant, Bronx, New York)

About a quarter of survey respondents answered that they went back to Korea for medical care because doctors in Korea had better ability than those in the United States. They gave two reasons that for this opinion: (1) doctors in Korea used more advanced methods and equipment than physicians in the United States, and (2) the academic credentials were more reliable in Korea than in the United States. First, the respondents identified that Korean doctors knew newer methods and more advanced technologies for medical care than the American doctors. Yang-Mi Kwon, who had a breast cancer surgery in Korea, found that the way of American doctor's surgery was out-dated than Korean doctor's, and that was one of the main reasons for her medical tours to Korea:

> I was diagnosed with a breast cancer in the US and had several follow-up examinations prior to a surgery. I found that American doctors' way of the operation was old-fashioned when I took a biopsy at a hospital in New Jersey. The American doctor used such a big needle to "dig up" my breast tissue. When I contacted my friend, who was a medical doctor in Korea, she told me that the American way was too brutal. That was the reason why I decided to go back to Korea for a breast cancer surgery. Once my doctor in Korea saw how American physicians' did a biopsy, he was surprised by American physicians' outdated operation methods. In Korea, nobody used that old method anymore. (Yang-Mi Kwon, 50, housewife, Palisades Park, New Jersey)

Second, some Korean informants expressed their doubts about the academic credentials of the US medical schools, not only for *Hanui* who practices *Hanbang*, but also for American doctors in general. Young-Chul

Doh, a 73-year-old male informant, emphasized that it is harder to get into the medical school in Korea than in the United States. Ji-Hye Kim also argued that American doctors were not as well educated as doctors in Korea:

> American doctors did not seem to be professional because of their academic credentials. In Korea, doctors had to study very hard to enter the medical school and receive their medical degrees. Not everybody can be a doctor in Korea; only a smart person can be a doctor. However, being a doctor is like getting a license in the US; anyone can be a doctor. I did not feel relieved when I saw a doctor in the US because their academic credentials were less reliable than in Korea. (Ji-Hye Kim, 26, employee at a Korean firm, Forest Hill, Queens)

While other reasons for medical tourism were pull factors, having no insurance in the United States was a strong push factor to Korean immigrants' medical tours to the home country. Nearly one-fifth of respondents indicated that having no insurance was the primary reason for their decision on medical tourism. Young-Ho Chung was an elderly man whose medical tourism was exclusively caused by his uninsured status in the United States. Except for not having health insurance in the United States, he had no other push factors to receive medical care in Korea; he spoke good English; he knew American culture well for working in the US Armed Forces in Korea over 30 years; he had two children in New Jersey who could help him to get to the hospital; He had good Korean network in the United States for being an elder of the Korean ethnic church. Only the financial issue caused by uninsured status was a problem for him to receive medical care in the United States, and that contributed to his medical tourism.

One's health insurance status was a complicated issue because it was related to age, occupation, legal status, and other factors. One thing noticeable about Korean immigrants' health insurance status was that it was closely related to their occupations. As reviewed in chapter 1, my survey data confirmed that self-employed Korean immigrants showed a much lower insurance rate than those employed. And this negative association was statistically significant. Not only self-employed Korean immigrants but also Korean immigrants who worked at a Korean firm showed a lower insurance rate than those who worked at a non-Korean firm or public sector. These results suggest that self-employed Koreans and Korean immigrant employees at Korean firms had fewer class resources and more financial barriers to the US healthcare. In fact, many self-employed informants reported that it was hard to see a doctor in the United States due to their uninsured status and long working hours. In chapter 4, the association among Korean immigrants' health insurance status, their employment status, and their decision on medical tours to the home country will be extensively examined using the survey data of all 507 respondents.

Another quarter of respondents (27/121 = 22.3%) gave other reasons for their medical tours to Korea. There were three other reasons, which were not associated with barriers to the US healthcare or other healthcare behaviors. The first was to get the second opinion from doctors in Korea. Kyung-Sook Baek, a middle-aged housewife with two children, visited Korea searching for a second opinion after her thyroid cancer diagnosis in the United States. Three years ago, she was diagnosed with thyroid cancer, and she had a surgery in the United States. Although the surgery was successful, she lost her voice as a side effect. Her American doctor told her to give up on recovering her voice. She was disappointed at his advice, but she did not give up her hope. Then, she suddenly remembered what her friend told her: "When you are diagnosed with cancer, you have to see different doctors for second, third, and fourth opinions." To get the second opinion, her sister in Korea made an appointment for her with a famous doctor at Samsung Medical Center. A second opinion from the Korean doctor was positive, and she had her voice back after several treatments.

The second reason was to receive treatments for diseases which were more prevalent among Koreans than Americans. Jung-Sook Lee and Kyung-Hee Kim were two medical tourists who wanted to receive treatments for diseases that were more common in Korea than in the United States. Since many Koreans suffer from certain diseases, they believed that frequent operations make expert doctors in these medical fields. An esophageal cancer was one of these diseases. According to Kyung-Hee Kim, an informant in her late 40s, esophageal cancer was more prevalent among Koreans, but not among Americans. Consequently, there were many Korean doctors who have operated esophageal cancer. However, it was difficult for her to find a doctor who has performed the surgery many times in the United States. That was the primary reason why she returned to Korea for a better and easier surgery when she found out that she was at the primary stage of esophageal cancer. Jung-Soon Lee, who had hepatitis B, also took a medical trip to the home country for a similar reason:

> I was diagnosed with hepatitis B about 30 years ago. Hepatitis B was a rare disease in the US, whereas Hepatitis A and C were more common among Americans. By contrast, it was quite a prevalent disease in Korea. That is the primary reason why I went back to Korea to see Dr. Kim, an expert of the liver at SNU hospital when I knew that I had hepatitis B. (Jung-Soon Lee, 67, fabric designer, Manhattan, New York)

Lastly, some Korean informants believed that Korean medical facilities and equipment were better and newer than American ones. They commonly complimented the facilities of Korean hospitals. Clean and fancy hospital buildings in Korea, which looked like "shopping malls," or "department stores," gave them a feeling of trust in receiving medical treatments there. Soo-Bin Kim, who worked as a dental technician in Flushing, went back to Korea for medical care because she thought that Korean doctors could discover any disease better than American doctors, as Korean hospitals did not hesitate to buy the best and newest medical equipment. Another informant, Eun-Jung Choi described that newest medical equipment was one of the primary reasons for her medical tours to the home country:

> Korean hospitals were incomparable to the US hospitals in terms of medical devices. Several years ago, I had a severe pain in my stomach. When I visited a doctor's office in the US, they just told me that I had a lump in my stomach. They did not specify where I had a lump in my stomach. However, when I saw a doctor in Korea for the same symptom a few months later, he pinpointed out a particular area at a certain membrane of my stomach where the lump was located in. Since my Korean doctor had the best and newest medical technologies, he discovered exactly where I had a problem with my stomach. (Eun-Jung Choi, 41, employee at a Korean firm, Flushing, Queens)

In summary, Korean immigrants' barriers to the US healthcare and their healthcare behaviors are highly associated. Considering all contributing factors, Table 3.7 shows a typology of Korean immigrants' coping strategies based on the two most influential barriers: (1) their insured status as an example of financial barriers, and (2) the level of personal barriers, such as language or cultural barriers. Although structural barriers, such as undocumented status or the number of Korean doctors, might be other important contributing factors, they are not included in Table 3.7 because they do not seem to be as dominant as financial and cultural barriers for Korean immigrants.

Korean immigrants with a low level of personal barriers and no US health insurance tend not to use any of three coping strategies discussed in this book. Rather, free clinics in the non-Korean community are their primary sources of medical care in the United States. They are likely to seek informal healthcare in the non-Korean community because no free clinic is provided by Korean community centers in the NY-NJ area due to liability issues. By contrast, Korean immigrants who have US health insurance and a low level of personal barriers are likely to see American doctors. This group is the least marginalized one. Doubly disadvantaged Korean immigrants with serious language or cultural barriers and uninsured status form the group that utilizes the three coping strategies most actively. On the other hand, if

**Table 3.7 Types of Coping Strategies Based on Barriers to Formal US Healthcare**

| *Level of Personal Barriers (e.g., Language or Cultural)* | *Financial Barrier (e.g., Health Insured Status in the United States)* | |
|---|---|---|
| | *Uninsured in the United States* | *Insured in the United States* |
| Low | • Go to free clinics in non-Korean community | • See American doctors<br>• The least marginalized group |
| High | • See co-ethnic doctors<br>• Use *Hanbang*<br>• Medical tours to the home country | • See co-ethnic doctors<br>• Medical tours to the home country |

insured Korean immigrants have a high level of personal barriers, they tend to see co-ethnic doctors in the United States or make frequent visits to Korea to receive treatment.

As explained earlier, Portes and associates (2012) pointed out several possible coping strategies based on the type of immigrant barriers to healthcare utilization in the United States. Their model seems to be applicable for Korean immigrants in most cases. The biggest difference between the two models is that Portes and associates considered medical tourism as a coping strategy mainly for recent immigrants, whereas Koreans who lived in the United States for a long time still actively use it as one of their strategies. This is likely because Korean immigrants maintain a high level of transnational ties with the home country (Min 2013; Noh, Kwak, and Han 2013), which encourages old-timers to visit the home country for medical care.

In this regard, chapter 4 focuses particularly on how other types of transnational ties (e.g., social, political, and cultural) are associated with Korean immigrants' medical tourism to the home country. Moreover, since reasons for medical tourism assessed in this chapter were based on the answers of Korean immigrants who only participated in medical tourism ($N = 121$), it was not possible to understand the contributing factors to all Korean immigrants' medical tourism decisions, although their responses were helpful to understand why they decided to take medical tours to Korea. To thoroughly examine major contributing factors, chapter 4 includes all survey respondents ($N = 507$) as well as my in-depth personal interviews with the participants of medical tourism ($N = 100$) and the nonparticipants of medical tourism ($N = 20$).

# *Chapter 4*

# Factors Contributing to Korean Immigrants' Medical Tourism

## TRANSNATIONAL TIES AS CONTRIBUTING FACTORS TO MEDICAL TOURISM

As mentioned in Introduction, immigrants' medical tourism does not stand alone. It is closely connected with other types of transnationalism: political, economic, social, cultural, and religious transnationalism. Moreover, as pointed out in chapter 3, Korean immigrants' high level of transnational ties with the home country is assumed to be influential on their medical tours to the home country. Thus, this section intends to examine how other types of transnationalism are correlated with Korean immigrants' decision on medical tourism.

### The Association between the Number of Visits to Korea and Medical Tourism

Before examining the relationship between medical tourism and other types of transnationalism, it is important to know the frequency of Korean immigrants' visit to Korea for any purpose as it represents the central aspect of their transnational ties with the home country. Moreover, it is likely to be strongly related to their medical tourism, which requires individuals' physical visit to the home country. The immigrants who visit their country of origin more often for any purpose are more likely to have medical care as well since they need a trip to the home country for it. Table 4.1 indicates the frequency of Korean immigrants' visit to Korea for any purpose. The majority (78%) of Korean immigrants had ever visited Korea for any reason since their migration to the United States, but still, a substantial proportion of them (22%) had never visited Korea since their immigration. These numbers were similar to what Min (2013) found earlier

**Table 4.1 Number of Visits to Korea Since Migration to the United States**

| *Number Visits to Korea* | N | % |
|---|---|---|
| Never visited | 112 | 22.1 |
| Once | 83 | 16.4 |
| 2–3 times | 132 | 26.0 |
| 4–8 times | 124 | 24.5 |
| 9 times or more | 56 | 11.0 |
| Total | 507 | 100.0 |

*Source*: Survey of 507 Korean immigrants in the NY-NJ area.

based on his survey in the NY-NJ area: about 85% of Korean immigrants have ever visited Korea and more than half of them (54%) have visited Korea three times or more often since their migration to the United States.

Old-timers who had lived in the United States for 20 years or longer had a greater propensity for visiting the home country than their newcomer counterparts, who had stayed in the United States less than 10 years. About one-tenth of old-timers and about a quarter of newcomers had never visited Korea since their migration to the United States. Perhaps newcomers would not have long enough time to visit the homeland due to their relatively shorter migration periods. Among Korean immigrants who had ever visited Korea ($N = 395$), about the one-fifth had visited their home country for just once. The vast majority of them had visited Korea twice or more.

Table 4.2 shows that the number of visits to Korea has a positive association with the number of medical tours to Korea. Certainly, those who had never visited Korea for any purpose did not take any medical tour to the home country. However, those who visited Korea more often for any purposes also had more medical tours to the home country. The positive and significant association between the number of visits to Korea and medical tourism was probably due to the fact that Korean immigrants' medical tours were often mixed with other purposes.

In fact, among 121 Korean immigrants who have ever participated in medical tourism, only 6.6% of them answered that the purpose of visiting the home country was exclusively for the medical purpose. The vast majority of Korean immigrant medical tourists answered that the reason for their visit to the home country was mixed with the medical and other purposes. Korean immigrants who had participated in medical tourism had other reasons, such as visiting family and friends (86.0%), sightseeing (14.9%), business purposes (9.9%), and visa-related issues (6.6%). About 3.3% of them reported that attending funerals or weddings in Korea was another reason for their visit to Korea, along with the medical purpose.

Based on the conversations with my informants, there were two groups of Korean immigrants who had visited Korea only for medical purposes. First,

**Table 4.2 Number of Medical Tours by the Number of Visits to Korea**

| | *Number of Visits to Korea for Any Reason* | | | |
|---|---|---|---|---|
| *Number of Medical Tours* | *None* | *1–3 Times* | *4 Times or More* | *Total* |
| None | 112 (100.0%) | 160 (74.4%) | 115 (63.9%) | 386 (76.1%) |
| Once | 0 (0%) | 32 (14.9%) | 18 (10.0%) | 51 (10.1%) |
| Twice or more | 0 (0%) | 23 (10.7%) | 47 (26.1%) | 70 (13.8%) |
| Total | 112 (100.0%) | 215 (100.0%) | 180 (100.0%) | 507 (100.0%) |

$\chi^2$ (4, $N$ = 507) = 62.43, $p$ = < .001/ gamma = .57.
*Source*: Survey of 507 Korean immigrants in the NY-NJ area.

some informants immediately went back to the home country for a major surgery after they were diagnosed with a serious disease (e.g., cancer) in the United States. For example, Jung-Hoon Lee, a middle-aged taxi driver in Queens, went back to Korea about five years ago once he found that he had a thyroid cancer. Yang-Mi Kwon was another person who went back to Korea right after she knew that she had a breast cancer in 2006. Korean immigrants who belong to the first type commonly wanted to "have a knife on their body" in the home country than in the United States because as an ethnic minority they were afraid of receiving paid less attention by non-Korean doctors in the United States. Sung-Ho Lim indeed had a medical tour to Korea for this reason, fear of being an experimental subject during the surgery by non-Korean doctors:

> As an Asian immigrant, I often experience racial discrimination in the US. I suspected that American doctors used us as guinea pigs here. Last year, I needed to get rid of skin adhesion near my ear, and I wanted to go back to Korea because it was a surgery that puts a knife on my body. I did not want to do it here because I had a stereotype for them to pay less attention to Asian patients. They would do their best to White Americans, but not to us, Asians. (Sung-Ho Lim, 58, taxi driver, Bayside, Queens)

The second group includes Korean immigrants those who needed follow-up treatments for the prior surgeries which had been operated in Korea. For example, Hyun-Jung Choi, a 37-year-old female accountant, received a shoulder surgery in 2005 in Suwon, Korea. Since she preferred to see the same doctor who operated her surgery before, she went back to Korea in 2006 and 2013 for following checkups and treatments for her shoulder. Young-Ho Kim and Joong-Soo Lim were two elderly Korean immigrants who took medical tours for follow-up treatments of their prior surgeries operated in Korea. Young-Ho, a 78-year-old man who had lived in the United States for more than 40 years, visited Korea annually for the last couple of years. Since he began his first dental implant procedure in Korea, he has visited Korea for follow-up treatments and another implant per each visit. Joong-Soo, a 76-year-old man, also visited Korea annually for the last three years to meet the doctor who performed his heart surgery in the past. During each visit, the doctor checked up if his heart functioned properly. He could see a doctor in the United States for the follow-up of his surgery, but he wanted to be examined by the doctor who had conducted his surgery because he considered that doctor would know his body better than an unfamiliar doctor in the United States.

In chapter 1, I speculated that the members of a *Kirogi* family, a new form of transnational family that consist of a mother and children staying in the United States and a father staying in Korea, would have a greater tendency to take medical tours to Korea because they are likely to visit Korea more often than non-transnational family members. Unfortunately, the proportion of a *Kirogi* family was not high among my Korean informants as only 12 of 507 (2.4%) survey respondents answered that they had spouses in Korea. The vast majority of them were women in their 40s and 50s and had children. Most of them were newcomers who have lived in the United States less than ten years, supposedly, for their children's education. As expected, they showed a much higher percentage of taking medical tours to the home country than those who did not have spouses in Korea. During in-depth personal interviews, two *Kirogi* mothers indicated their frequent medical tours because they had to go back to Korea regularly to take care of the left ones: *Kirogi* fathers. These *Kirogi* mothers showed a high degree of transnational lives: they have lived six months in the United States and another six months in Korea. Due to their frequent visits to Korea and extended stay there, they did not buy US health insurance and used Korea as the main place for their medical care.

## Social Transnationalism and Medical Tourism

In Introduction, I pointed out six areas of transnationalism that are relevant to immigrants—political, economic, social, cultural, religious, and medical. This section and the following section intend to examine the connection between and among medical transnationalism and other types of transnationalism. To measure the level of Korean immigrants' social transnational ties with the home country, I asked if they have any relatives in Korea and, if so, how often they contacted them. There were four possible different types of relatives in Korea that the survey respondents could choose: parents, siblings, spouse, and children. About a quarter had no relative in Korea. Slightly more than half had siblings, and about a half had parents in Korea. As indicated in the earlier section, only a few respondents had spouses in Korea. The elderly Korean immigrants were less likely to have any relatives in Korea probably because their parents were most likely to be passed away. Moreover, most of them had their children in the United States rather than in Korea.

The following tables indicate that Korean immigrants' social transnational ties with the home country are highly associated with their medical tourism experience. First, Table 4.3 shows that Korean immigrants who have relatives in Korea visited the home country more frequently for medical tourism. For example, about 91% of Korean immigrants who have no relatives in Korea have never taken medical tours to the home country. By contrast, more than a quarter of Korean immigrants who have any relatives in Korea have taken medical tours to the home country once or more. Moreover, the strength of the positive association between the number of medical tourism visits and having any relatives in Korea was strong.

Having any relatives in Korea was a mediating factor to the relationship between visiting Korea and taking medical tours to Korea. Most of all, Korean immigrants who had any relatives in Korea were more likely to visit the homeland. And those who visited Korea more often were more likely to take medical tours to the home country. It is difficult to determine whether having relatives *promoted* Korean immigrants' medical tours to Korea because the chi-squared test does not indicate the causality of association. However, many interviewees indicated that having relatives in Korea made it much easier for them to visit Korea for either general or medical purposes because they could stay with their relatives and avoid paying for a hotel or other lodging accommodations. One interviewee in her late 30s told me that having a place to stay for free influenced her decision to get her OB/GYN treatments in Korea.

In fact, the majority of non-medical tourists complained that having no relatives in the home country strongly influenced their decision not to take medical tours because they needed to pay for a hotel in Korea. For example, Min-Ho Park, a middle-aged man who has been in the United States for almost 20 years, had no relatives in Korea because all of his relatives migrated to the United States. Additionally, he married a US-born second-generation Korean woman, so he did not have any in-laws in Korea either. He said that since he did not have any relatives in Korea, he would need to stay at a hotel. Even if he wanted to go to Korea for medical tourism, he was unwilling to pay extra money for hotel accommodations.

**Table 4.3 Number of Medical Tours by Having Any Relatives in Korea**

| *Number of Medical Tours* | *Number of Relatives in Korea* | | |
|---|---|---|---|
| | *No Relative* | *Any Relatives* | *Total* |
| None | 119 (90.8%) | 267 (71.0%) | 386 (76.1%) |
| Once | 9 (6.9%) | 42 (11.2%) | 51 (10.1%) |
| Twice or more | 3 (2.3%) | 67 (17.8%) | 70 (13.8%) |
| Total | 131 (100.0%) | 376 (100.0%) | 507 (100.0%) |

$\chi^2$ (2, $N$ = 507) = 23.77, $p$ = < .001/ gamma = .61.

*Source*: Survey of 507 Korean immigrants in the NY-NJ area.

Not only having any relatives but also the frequency of contacting them is also important as a type of social transnational ties. Not surprisingly, there was a positive association between frequent contact with relatives and medical tourism. Basch, Schiller, and Blanc (1994) argued that modern communication technologies have promoted transnationalism. This indeed seems to be the case for the Korean immigrants, as email, cheaper or even free international phone service, texting, video calling, and Kakaotalk (a popular Korean mobile application that offers free message service) have helped Korean immigrants maintain much easier and more frequent contacts with relatives in Korea, thus, facilitating social transnational ties.

Korean immigrants who had spouses in the home country showed the most frequent contacts than those who had any other types of relatives in Korea. However, as noticed earlier, the number of individuals who had spouses in Korea, supposedly *Kirogi* mothers, was very small. Those who had parents in Korea also showed frequent contacts, but not as much as those who had spouses. By contrast, having siblings or children in Korea was not associated with the number of contacts.

Previously, Noh, Kwak, and Han (2013) have found that Korean immigrants in Canada had strong social transnational ties with the home country; more than half of them have at least one parent in Korea, and about 80% of them have talked to them via telephone. Moreover, they have found that young and recent immigrants showed stronger social transnational ties than their older and old-timer counterparts. Their findings were similar to what I found with my own survey data. First, young Korean immigrants in the NY-NJ area showed more frequent contacts with their relatives in Korea than their elderly counterparts. About two-thirds of non-elderly Korean immigrants had contacted their relatives in Korea a few times a month or more frequent, whereas only about half of elderly Koreans had done so. This was probably because elderly Korean immigrants tended to have a fewer number of relatives in Korea as their parents were likely to be dead and as their children were likely to stay in the United States with them. Second, newcomers had contacted their relatives in Korea more frequently than their old-timer counterparts. About 90% of newcomers who had lived in the United States less than ten years had contacted their relatives a few times a month or more frequently. About two-thirds of them had contacted their relatives every week or more frequently. By contrast, about half of old-timers who had lived in the United States for more than 20 years had contacted their relatives a few times a month or more frequently. About 18% had weekly based or more frequent contacts with their relatives in Korea.

Table 4.4 shows that people who contacted their relatives in Korea more frequently are more likely to take medical tours to the home country. About 17% of Korean immigrants who contacted their relatives in Korea a few times

**Table 4.4 Number of Medical Tours by Contacting with Relatives in Korea**

| | *Frequency of Contacts with Relatives in Korea* | | | |
|---|---|---|---|---|
| *Number of Medical Tours* | *Less Than a Few Times a Month* | *A Few Times a Month* | *Every Week or More Frequently* | *Total* |
| None | 88 (83.8%) | 91 (72.8%) | 88 (60.3%) | 267 (71.0%) |
| Once | 9 (8.6%) | 14 (11.2%) | 19 (13.0%) | 42 (11.2%) |
| Twice or more | 8 (7.6%) | 20 (16.0%) | 39 (26.7%) | 67 (17.8%) |
| Total[1] | 105 (100.0%) | 125 (100.0%) | 146 (100.0%) | 376 (100.0%) |

[1]This analysis includes Korean immigrants who have any relatives in Korea ($N = 376$).
$\chi^2$ (4, $N = 376$) = 18.77, $p < .01$/ gamma = .36.
*Source*: Survey of 507 Korean immigrants in the NY-NJ area.

a year had at least one medical tourism experience. More than a quarter of Koreans who kept in touch with their relatives in Korea a few times a month had engaged in medical tourism to the home country. Those who contacted their relatives every week or more frequently showed the highest tendency of taking medical tours to Korea (39.7%); 13% took medical tours once, and 26.7% took medical tours twice or more. Contacting their relatives in Korea also affected Korean immigrants' arrangement of medical tourism. I examine that in chapter 5 as this chapter focuses on social transnational ties as the contributing factor to the decision, rather than the arrangement, of Korean immigrants' medical tourism.

In chapter 1, I analyzed the 2009–2011 ACS data and found that Korean immigrants' educational level was high in general, and the variation of their educational level was not wide. I suspected any association between the educational level and medical tourism—either positive or negative—because more educated immigrants might have more opportunities to visit the home country using more economic resource through their higher education or they might have fewer chances due to their better social networks in the United States through their higher human capital. However, the educational level itself was not significantly associated with Korean immigrants' medical tours. Yet, interestingly, the in-depth interviews revealed that respondents' college education often strengthened their social transnational ties with the home country, playing a mediating factor to their decisions to engage in medical tourism. There were several informants who noted that transnational events organized by their alma maters in Korea influenced their medical tourism. Five interviewees said that they went to university hospitals that were affiliated with the universities where they graduated. Often, alumni associations invited overseas alumni to Korea for several events, such as a homecoming day. Many of these alumni were eligible for discounted medical bills from the university-affiliated hospitals. These types of financial benefits through social transnational ties were influential factors to engaging in medical tourism. For instance, Yang-Hoon Choi, a 66-year-old man, visited Konkuk

University Hospital, which was affiliated with his alma mater. Konkuk University Hospital offered him a 30% discounted medical bill and a 20% discounted price for his wife, thus, he and his wife took medical tours to Korea. For Jae-Yong Ryu, another interviewee, strong emotional attachments to his alma mater was another important issue. In his case, medical tourism was deeply associated with an invitation from the alumni association of his alma mater in Korea:

> When I visited Korea last time, I went to Chung-Ang University Hospital and received a regular checkup because I graduated from Chung-Ang University. The central alumni association of Chung-Ang University in Korea invited all the overseas alumni members. About 40 of us, the alumni members from the US, stayed in the university dorm. For three days and four nights, we went sightseeing and attended several university events. The alumni association offered a special rate for a regular checkup at Chung-Ang University hospital for people who wanted to receive it. About half of us had a regular checkup. The alumni association provided lodging at the dorm for extra days for people who needed a longer stay for their checkup. I felt that the university hospital gave us an extra and special care because we were the alumni. Moreover, I felt very comfortable at the hospital because I had strong emotional attachments to the University. (Jae-Yong Ryu, 61, business owner, Fort Lee, New Jersey)

## Political, Economic, and Cultural Transnationalism and Medical Tourism

In addition to social transnationalism, other types of transnational ties with the home country were related to Korean immigrants' medical tourism to the home country, but not as much as social transnational ties. As I reviewed in chapter 1, Korean immigrants in Canada showed weak political transnational ties with the home country (Noh, Kwak, and Han 2013). My survey data and in-depth personal interviews also indicated that Korean immigrants in the NY-NJ area had a low degree of political transnational ties with the homeland. Only two informants had political transnational ties with the home country by participating in the political organization to support certain politicians. However, their political transnational ties were not related to their medical tours to the home country.

Interestingly, three elderly interviewees reported that their political transnational ties were closely connected to their medical tourism. In 2010, the Korean government revised the Nationality Act, and it strongly influenced Korean immigrants' political transnational ties to the home country. Before 2010, Korean immigrants who wanted to attain dual nationality had to give up the other nationality to recover the Korean nationality. However, the revised Article 9 of the Nationality Act states: "A person who had been residing in a foreign country and entered Korea for permanent residency at the age of 65 or older has attained permission for reinstatement of nationality." Thus, those who qualify this condition do not need to renounce a foreign nationality to regain their Korean nationality. After their reinstatement of Korean nationality, they have to fulfill the national obligation of tax payment and the Korean national health insurance payment. Also, they can exercise the right to vote if they register as residents with the Korean government. Since the United States approves multiple nationalities, they can still receive social security benefits, pension, Medicare, or other welfares from the United States. Recently in 2014, ten members of the National Assembly proposed a revised law that allows overseas Koreans who are 45 years old or older apply for dual nationality (Shin 2014).

Dual nationality has promoted some elderly Korean immigrants' medical tours to the home country because it has allowed them to have easier access to the Korean national health insurance. Ho-Sang Park, a 70-year-old man who recently received dual nationality, described his experience:

> As a dual citizen of the US and Korea, it became easier for me to visit the home country. I also have Korean national health insurance now. Once you became a dual citizen, you could be fully covered by health insurance with only about 90 dollars a month in Korea. I also have Medicare in the US, but I still visit Korea to see a doctor. If I saw a doctor in the US, about 100 dollars would be deducted from social. In Korea, the co-pay was only three or four dollars with the national insurance. After recovering my Korean nationality, I also felt more attached to my home country. (Ho-Sang Park, 70, retired, Palisades Park, New Jersey)

My interview with another Korean senior citizen revealed how political transnational ties, as well as economic transnational ties, were connected to his medical tourism experience:

> I came to the US in 1991 and ran a dry cleaning store before my retirement. I visited Korea last year to recover my Korean citizenship, still maintaining the US citizenship. Last year, I read a local Korean newspaper which was published in New Jersey, and the article reported that Korean immigrants who were older than 65 years could apply for the dual citizenship. Actually, I applied for the dual citizenship not for the medical purpose, but for the economic purpose. I had an apartment in Seoul, which I bought before migration to the US and wanted to sell it. But the property tax rate was about 70% as an American citizen. After being a dual citizen of two countries, I sold the apartment with lower tax rates. Moreover, I had more chances to visit Korea for the medical purpose. I already had a checkup and dental treatments there because I visited there more often. (Sang-Chul Choi, 73, retired, Palisades Park, New Jersey)

Cultural transnational ties had a mild effect on Korean immigrants' medical tourism. Only two informants said that advertisements in a Korean newspaper published in the NY-NJ area contributed to their decision to engage in medical tourism. This is probably because the travel agencies' passive strategies to attract overseas Koreans as indicated in chapter 2. Rather, cultural transnationalism influenced the aftereffects of their medical tourism, which will be discussed in chapter 5. Regarding the association between religious transnational ties and medical tourism, three informants who had Won Buddhism as their religion reported that they went to Wonkwang University Hospital in Korea, which was affiliated with Won Buddhism. However, other than them, there were no informants whose medical tourism was related to their religious transnational ties with the home country.

## HEALTH INSURANCE STATUS AS A CONTRIBUTING FACTOR TO MEDICAL TOURISM

Previous studies found the lack of health insurance was one of the major contributing factors to immigrants' medical tourism because uninsured immigrants tended to have more difficulties receiving medical care in the United States (Brown 2008; Landeck and Garza 2003). In chapter 1, analyzing the 2009–2011 ACS data, I presented that foreign-born Koreans had a lower insurance rates than their native-born non-Hispanic whites and US-born Koreans counterparts. When I asked all survey respondents ($N = 507$) about their health insurance status, nearly 30% had no health insurance in the United States. I assumed that uninsured Korean immigrants would show a higher chance of taking medical tours to the home country than their insured counterparts due to more financial barriers to access to US healthcare.

However, Table 4.5 shows that the association between health insurance status and medical tourism was statistically not significant. Seventy-seven percent of uninsured and 76% of insured Korean immigrants did not participate in medical tourism. Certainly, for most uninsured Korean immigrants, the home country was often the *ultimate* place of medical care. Due to the expensive medical costs in the United States without health insurance, most of them had no choice but to visit the home country for medical treatment. In particular, medical tours to the home country was an excellent option for middle-aged Korean immigrants who were retired but not yet eligible for Medicare. The home country was the *ultimate* place of medical care when their US health insurance through their job had been terminated with their retirement and when they were not yet qualified for Medicare because they were younger than 65 years old.

There are two reasons for this insignificant relationship between Korean immigrants' health insurance status and their medical tours to the home

**Table 4.5 Number of Medical Tours by Health Insurance Status**

| *Number of Medical Tours* | *Health Insurance Status* | | |
|---|---|---|---|
| | *Not Insured* | *Insured* | *Total* |
| None | 114 (77.0%) | 272 (75.8%) | 386 (76.1%) |
| Once | 13 (8.8%) | 38 (10.6%) | 51 (10.1%) |
| Twice or more | 21 (14.2%) | 49 (13.6%) | 70 (13.8%) |
| Total | 148 (100.0%) | 359 (100.0%) | 507 (100.0%) |

$\chi^2$ (2, *N* = 507) = 0.38, *p* > .05.
*Source*: Survey of 507 Korean immigrants in the NY-NJ area.

country. It is difficult to explain these reasons by quantitative analysis of the survey data. However, fortunately, my in-depth personal interviews with Korean immigrant medical tourists found an interesting phenomenon regarding this insignificant association.

On the one hand, Korean immigrants who had the US health insurance still took medical tours to the home country. There were four types of Korean immigrants who took medical tours despite having health insurance in the United States: (1) those who viewed Korea as an *alternative* option for medical care depending on their needs, (2) those who used Korea as a *supplementary* place of medical care, (3) those who considered Korea as a *secure* place of medical care due to the complicated nature of healthcare in the United States, and (4) those who viewed Korea as a *superior* place for medical care. Interestingly, the main reasons for their medical tourism and the ways of using the home country as the place of medical care were different across the four groups of these insured Korean immigrants.

The first type was those who visited Korea for mixed purposes with their US health insurance. For them, Korea was an *alternative* place where they might or might not get medical care depending on their situation. According to my survey, only 6.6% of Korean immigrant medical tourists visited Korea only for medical purposes. The vast majority of other Korean immigrant medical tourists visited Korea partly for medical and partly for other purposes, such as visiting family and friends or taking business trips. Eun-Ji Kim, a middle-aged employee at a Korean firm in the United States, explained that her regular visits to Korea contributed to her medical tours to the home country although she had US health insurance: "I had an excellent health insurance through my job, but I tried not to see a doctor in the United States unless it was an urgent situation. As I have visited Korea regularly and annually to see my family, I could solve all my health issues in Korea. The medical processes were less complicated, and the medical costs were cheaper there." Hyun-Woo Park, a middle-aged businessman, visited Korea regularly, primarily for business purposes. He visited Korea at least twice a year and, like Eun-Ji Kim, he used Korea as an *alternative* place of medical care. Since Korea provided cheaper medical treatments for him, he even canceled his US health insurance. In this case, the home country became an *ultimate* place of medical care rather than an *alternative* place. Korean immigrants who belong to this first type commonly reported that faster medical processes in Korea was the primary reason for their medical tourism.

The second type was those who still visited Korea for medical care because (1) their US health insurance did not cover optical or dental treatment or (2) because their US plans only offered limited coverage. For them, the home country was a *supplementary* place of medical care. They could have received optical or dental care in the United States, but cheaper medical costs in Korea was the biggest reason for their medical tourism, as they needed to pay more medical expenses for the same optical or dental treatments in the United States. Ji-Won Kim, an interviewee in her late 30s, had Lasik corrective eye surgery during her last visit to Korea. As an employee at a Korean-American firm, she had health insurance with good coverage for general medical care. However, her US insurance did not cover any optical treatments or surgeries. Although she received all of her other medical care in the United States, she visited Korea for optical treatments. Many other Korean immigrants in this supplemental category also frequently traveled to Korea to receive dental care. Hye-Young Kim, a middle-aged housewife, said that she had US health insurance with good coverage for general healthcare. For example, it only cost about 20 dollars for her to get an endoscopy with her US insurance. However, her plan did not cover any dental treatments, so whenever she visited Korea, she went to see a dentist there.

The second type also includes Korean immigrants whose US health insurance offered limited coverage, which contributed to the need to take medical tours to the homeland. For example, Soo-Jin Bang had a health insurance plan with very limited coverage. Thus, when she had a car accident in the United States, only a few physical therapy sessions were covered by her insurance. Since she felt that the total number of visits to the physical therapist was not enough, she visited Korea regularly to receive supplementary treatment:

> Medical tourism means supplementing treatments to me. When the numbers of treatment covered by my US insurance were not enough, I visited Korea for extra treatments. For example, I could have only one colonoscopy in every five years in the US. But, I wanted to have a colonoscopy every year. If I exceeded the limited numbers of treatments in the US, I needed to pay a huge amount of medical bill here. So, when I wanted to receive more examinations or treatments, I went back to Korea for that. (Soo-Jin Bang, 58, employee at a Korean firm, Fort Lee, New Jersey)

The third type was insured Korean immigrants who often went back to the home country due to the complicated and confusing nature of the US medical system. Most of all, complicated check-in procedures, long waiting time at the doctor's office, and having to make an appointment in advance made them use the home country as a *secure* place of medical care. Kyung-Hwa Chang, a 40-year-old woman who had been in the United States for nine years, preferred to go back to Korea for medical care even though she had Aetna insurance here. She felt that it was too inconvenient and complicated to call the doctor's office to check if they accept her insurance prior to her visits to the office. Also, she felt that making appointments, check-in and check-out procedures, the medical treatment itself, and waiting for results were too time-consuming in the United States. Another interviewee also expressed that complicated US medical processes influenced her to go back to Korea for medical treatment:

> One day, I had a deep scratch on my knee during exercise. I had health insurance, Blue Cross Blue Shield, but I needed to make several phone calls to the doctor's offices to check if they would accept my insurance. After several calls, I finally found a doctor who was willing to take mine, but that office was located too far from where I got injured. After going through all these complicated appointment-making processes in the US, I decided to go back to Korea for medical care. (Seo-Yoon Choi, 30, student, Woodside, Queens)

Additionally, the uncertainty of medical costs was another complication of the US healthcare system that some Korean immigrants wanted to avoid. Min-Joon Yoon, a 36-year-old man who worked at an American bank on Wall Street, pointed out that ambiguity regarding the price of medical procedures made him worried whenever he had any medical issues in the United States. A few years ago, he sprained his ankle while playing soccer. When he visited an orthopedic specialist, the doctors and nurses did not tell him how much he needed to pay for the treatment. A few months after his injury, to his surprise, he continued to receive a number of medical bills. After this experience, he became scared to see a doctor in the United States due to the uncertainty of pricing and medical bills. Thus, he tried to receive as many medical treatments as possible whenever he visited Korea. Another interviewee drew an analogy between paying medical bills and buying products in the United States:

> The US hospitals had such a complicated system, and that did not make any sense. For example, we purchased a product after checking its price. However, we could not know the amount of the expected medical treatments before going through it. Whenever I asked the expected price of the medical care, the receptionist or the doctor said that they could not tell it because it should be negotiated with the insurance company first. (Ji-Hyun Choi, 40, housewife, Flushing, Queens)

The last type was insured Korean immigrants who had better personal connections with medical doctors in Korea. For them, the home country was a *superior* place of medical care, as it provided better quality medical services and treatments through better social networks. For example, Min-Sik Choi was an old-timer Korean immigrant who migrated to the United States 35 years ago. Although he had a US health insurance plan with good coverage, he still visited Korea for medical treatment because his youngest sister was a doctor there. Another interviewee described how her higher level of social networks in Korea compared to the United States pushed her to go back to Korea despite her US health insurance:

> Although I was insured, I felt that there was a limitation for me to search and meet the noted doctors with excellent skills in the US. Maybe there were better physicians in the US. However, as an immigrant, I had no chance to meet them. In Korea, I had relatives who were doctors, so I had better networks to search and meet the noted doctors. That was the main reason for my medical tourism. (Ja-Kyung Park, 47, housewife, Palisades Park, New Jersey)

On the other hand, many uninsured Korean immigrants were not able to go back to Korea for medical tourism. There was a mediating factor to the association between Korean immigrants' health insurance status and medical tourism: their self-employment status. Self-employed Korean immigrants, who were more likely to be uninsured and thus, assumed to be more likely to take medical tours, could not visit Korea for medical purposes for several reasons. As previously mentioned in chapter 1, Korean immigrants were highly concentrated in the ethnic economy either as business owners or employees (Min 1984, 1990, and 2008; Min and Bozorgmehr 2003; Yoon 1991), and self-employed Koreans and the employees of small co-ethnic businesses were less likely to have insurance coverage than those in the public sector or the non-Korean private sector (Ryu, Young, and Park 2001). Thus, I hypothesized that self-employed Koreans would be more likely to go back to Korea to get medical care, assuming that they had less access to US healthcare due to their lower rates of having health insurance. My survey data also confirmed that self-employed Koreans had a lower insurance rate (57.0%) than their non-self-employed counterparts (73.6%).

However, it turned out that long working hours and the obligation to their stores hindered them from visiting their home country for medical and other purposes. Sang-Il Cha, a middle-aged self-employed man, mentioned that he had visited Korea just once (for his father's funeral) since migrating to the United States in the 1990s. Since he had his own business and needed to work all day and every day, including the weekends, it was impossible for him to visit Korea. Jeong-Sook Yoon, another entrepreneur who runs a laundry in New Jersey, told me that starting up a business totally changed her life, including her insured status and her chance of visiting Korea:

> I had visited Korea only three times in last 28 years. The last visit was about 17 years ago before having my own business. Before starting up my laundry, I had health insurance through my job. Now, as an entrepreneur, I have no insurance and no family doctor. Since I am not insured now, I would love to go to Korea to receive a regular checkup and other medical treatments. However, I do not have any personal time as an owner of a store. Time is so important us, like who have their own businesses. (Jeong-Sook Yoon, 55, laundry owner, Palisades Park, New Jersey)

However, self-employed Korean immigrants were not the only ones who could not take medical tours to Korea despite their low rate of having health insurance. Employees of small co-ethnic businesses, many of whom are recent and young Korean immigrants, also lack health insurance coverage. As indicated in the earlier chapters of this book, they showed a lower insurance rate than those who work in the public sector or at a non-Korean firm. However, they have difficulty traveling to Korea because they typically have trouble affording travel expenses. In personal interviews, a few employees at a Korean firm indicated that it was hard for them to visit Korea for medical and other purposes because they could not afford travel expenses. Sang-Hoon Choi, an employee at a small Korean-owned store in Flushing, described himself as a dayfly as he has lived from hand to mouth. During his 20 years in the United States, he has only visited Korea once, to attend his father's funeral. Since his Korean employer only paid him minimum wage without any paid vacation, he could barely make ends meet with his salary. Consequently, although he wanted to receive a medical checkup in Korea, taking medical tours to the home country was just a "pie in the sky."

## TEMPORARY RESIDENCE STATUS AS A CONTRIBUTING FACTOR TO MEDICAL TOURISM

In chapter 1, I pointed out that Korean immigrants' structural barriers to the healthcare in the United States were not considered as much as other types of barriers because they were considered to be less undocumented than Latino or Chinese immigrants. Yet, their legal status was found to be one of the most critical structural barriers to their medical tourism because undocumented Korean immigrants could not come back to the United States after getting medical treatments in the home country. Legal status was a very sensitive issue among immigrants, especially among the undocumented or people who temporarily stayed in the United States. Thus, some Korean immigrants were not willing to disclose their past and current legal status in the United States, and only about half of the survey respondents (264 out of 507) answered the question of their legal status. The survey respondents could choose the following five options: (1) temporary visa (e.g., student visa, visiting scholar and intern), (2) working visa (e.g., employees of Korean or US firms), (3) a permanent resident, (4) a naturalized citizen, and (5) other. About 5% of respondents chose the last category, and I presumed that they are most likely to be undocumented. Slightly more than 10% of survey respondents (11.0%) had a temporary visa, and 4.2% of them had a working visa. For the analysis of this section, I combined three types of Koreans (1) those who had a temporary visa, (2) those who had a working visa, and (3) those who had indicated his or her visa status as other, calling them as temporary residents. About one-third of the survey respondents were permanent residents, and nearly half of them (48.5%) were the US citizens.

During the in-depth personal interviews, some Korean immigrants voluntarily disclosed their undocumented status and explained how it influenced their medical tours to the home country. As expected, undocumented Korean immigrants or those who had complicated visa issues were not able to take medical tours to Korea. In fact, they could not visit the home country for any purposes because they were afraid of not coming back to the United States after visiting the home country. For example, a middle-aged male interviewee, who was unemployed and looking for a job, could not go back to Korea for the medical purpose due to his complicated legal status. Until a few months ago, he had maintained a working visa (H1B). But at the time of the interview, he was staying in the United States illegally. Due to his layoff, he did not have health insurance in the United States anymore. He wanted to go back to Korea when he was sick, but he could not visit Korea for the medical purpose or for any other purposes because he knew that he could not come back again once he left the United States.

Some Koreans discussed how their changed legal status influenced their decision on medical tour. Jung-Ae Kim, a 58-year-old housewife in Palisade Park, had wanted to go back to Korea for medical treatments because she had not been insured since her migration to the United States in the late 1990s. However, because of her undocumented status, she could not visit Korea for 11 years until she became a permanent resident. Finally, after recovering her legal status, she visited Korea twice for dental treatments and regular checkups. Another interviewee, Ok-Ja Jin, a 69-year-old retired woman, also indicated that her changed legal status contributed to her medical tourism experience:

> I have been in the US for 15 years. But until recently, my legal status did not allow me to go back to Korea. Five years ago, I was diagnosed with a uterine

myoma. I wanted to go back to Korea so badly to get a surgery due to the convenience of hospitalization processes in Korea. However, I could not go back because I was undocumented back then. So, I received surgery in the United States. A few years later, I received a green card. After then, I regularly went back to Korea every two years to get medical care. (Ok-Ja Jin, 69, retired, Fort Lee, New Jersey)

To examine the association between Korean immigrants' temporary resident status and the number of their medical tourism, I only included survey respondents who verified their legal status ($N = 264$). Thus, there were some limitations of this analysis because about half of the respondents who did not answer their legal status were excluded in this analysis. I assumed that they were likely to be undocumented or to have complicated visa issues. Also, some respondents, especially undocumented Korean immigrants, might give a false answer about their legal status. Despite these limitations, Table 4.6 indicates that the association between Korean immigrants' legal status and their medical tourism experience was statistically significant. As expected, temporary residents (40%) showed a higher percent of taking medical tours to Korea than their permanent residents (27%) or the US citizen counterparts (16%). In particular, a quarter (25%) of temporary residents took medical tours twice or more, whereas only 8.6% of Korean immigrants with the US nationality experienced two or more medical tourism to the home country.

There seem to be three factors to the association between Korean immigrants' temporary resident status and medical tourism: (1) the US health insurance, (2) the degree of transnational ties with the home country, and (3) the level of assimilation into the US society. First, Korean immigrants who stayed in the United States temporarily with student or working visas were less likely to be insured in the United States. Moreover, even if they had health insurance in the United States, they were more likely to have limited or minimal coverage. Although it was not shown in the table, my survey data confirmed the negative association between being temporary residents and

**Table 4.6 Number of Medical Tours by Legal Status**

| | *Legal Status* | | | |
|---|---|---|---|---|
| *Number of Medical Tours* | *Temporary Residents* | *Permanent Residents* | *US Citizens* | *Total* |
| None | 31 (59.6%) | 61 (72.6%) | 107 (83.6%) | 199 (75.4%) |
| Once | 8 (15.4%) | 6 (7.2%) | 10 (7.8%) | 24 (9.1%) |
| Twice or more | 13 (25.0%) | 17 (20.2%) | 11 (8.6%) | 41 (15.5%) |
| Total[1] | 52 (100.0%) | 84 (100.0%) | 128 (100.0%) | 264 (100.0%) |

[1]This analysis includes Korean immigrants who indicated their legal status ($N = 264$).
$\chi^2$ (4, $N = 264$) = 13.96, $p < .01$.
*Source*: Survey of 507 Korean immigrants in the NY-NJ area.

having health insurance in the United States. There are several reasons why temporary residents had a lower insurance rate than permanent residents or US citizens. As temporary residents, Korean immigrants cannot receive any public health insurance services such as Medicare or Medicaid. Moreover, they are likely to have less stable employment status due to their visa status.

Second, Korean immigrants who were temporary residents showed a much higher level of transnational ties with the home country than permanent residents or the US citizens. In particular, international students tended to take medical tours to the home country more often. This was due to their higher level of transnational social ties with the home country as they could go back to Korea during summer or winter vacations. Since they go back home during the break by any means, going to see a doctor in Korea was often their primary choice of healthcare. One female international student described:

> Every summer, I went back to Korea and had a regular checkup. I received dental care there too because getting a dental treatment was very expensive here with my student insurance. Also, my copay was too expensive here, and I could not afford it whenever I visit the doctor's office. So, when I was sick during the semester in the United States, I just took some painkillers. Then once the break began, I left for Korea and received medical treatments there. My regular visits to Korea during the vacation and expensive co-pay were important factors to my medical tourism. (Hye-Sil Kim, 25, student, Manhattan, New York)

Another international student stated that his regular visits to Korea during the summer or winter vacation contributed to his medical tourism:

> For many reasons, such as language problem and high medical cost in the United States, I did not go to see a doctor here. Since I visited Korea during the summer or winter breaks anyway, I usually tried to tolerate pain as much as possible when I was sick here. Recently, I had severe tooth pain. I knew a good dentist who attended my church in Flushing. But, I endured pain during the semester and then went home to see a dentist when the summer break began. (Tae-Wook Han, 24, student, Flushing, Queens)

Not only international students but also employees at big Korean firms also revealed strong transnational ties with the home country. Some of them had frequent business trips to Korea as they worked at Korean firms based in the United States. When they visited Korea for the business purpose, they often received medical care there. For example, Moon-Soo was a 36-year-old employee at a Korean securities company in Manhattan. His company in Korea sent him to the Manhattan office so that he could work there and earn an Executive MBA degree at Columbia Business School. During his two years of stay in the United States, he visited Korea twice for business meetings in Korea. He extended his stay in Korea so that he could receive dental treatments and a checkup at Korean hospitals.

Lastly, assimilation into the US society mediated the association between the temporary residence status and medical tourism. In general, temporary residents were less assimilated into the US society than permanent residents or the US citizens because they had lived in the United States for a shorter time period. Less assimilated immigrants would show a higher preference to take medical tours to the home country rather than to receive medical care in the United States due to language barriers or cultural affinity to the home country. Table 4.7 supports this hypothesis by showing a negative association between years spent in the United States and medical tourism experience among Korean immigrants. Newcomers who have lived in the United States less than 10 years showed a higher tendency of taking medical tourism. Almost 40% had experienced at least one medical tourism. By contrast, old-timers who have resided in the United States for more than 20 years showed the lowest rate of experiencing medical tourism. Only 5.4% of them had taken a medical tour once, and about 9.2% of them took two or more medical tours to the home country.

The personal interviews with Korean immigrant medical tourists also confirmed this pattern; as they assimilated into the American society more, they received medical care in the United States than went back to the home country for medical care. Jae-Joon Lim, a 37-year-old government officer, said that he took medical tours frequently during his early migration period:

> I have visited Korea seven times since I migrated to the United States in 2000. But my medical tours to Korea happened mostly at the beginning of my life in America. Back in the early 2000s, I even maintained my Korean national health insurance so that I could receive medical care whenever I went back to see my parents. After becoming a permanent resident, I did not go to hospitals in Korea anymore because I felt that I needed to see a doctor here to settle down. As I have lived here longer, I have become more assimilated into the American society. As a permanent resident, it was the time to solve all my medical issues here rather than going back to Korea. (Jae-Joon Lim, 37, government officer, Manhattan, New York)

**Table 4.7 Number of Medical Tours by the Years in the United States**

| | *Years in the United States* | | | |
|---|---|---|---|---|
| *Number of Medical Tours* | *1–9 Years* | *10–19 Years* | *20 Years or Longer* | *Total* |
| None | 72 (61.0%) | 139 (75.5%) | 175 (85.4%) | 386 (76.1%) |
| Once | 17 (14.4%) | 23 (12.5%) | 11 (5.4%) | 51 (10.1%) |
| Twice or more | 29 (24.6%) | 22 (12.0%) | 19 (9.2%) | 70 (13.8%) |
| Total | 118 (100.0%) | 184 (100.0%) | 205 (100.0%) | 507 (100.0%) |

$\chi^2$ (4, $N$ = 507) = 27.06, $p < .001$/ gamma = –.375.
*Source*: Survey of 507 Korean immigrants in the NY-NJ area.

Jae-Joon also said that his preference for Korean doctors had been changed to non-Korean doctors in the United States due to his changed legal status and his greater assimilation into the US society:

> When I first arrived in the United States, I was an international student. Back then, I strongly preferred to go back to Korea to see a Korean doctor. I tried to endure pain as much as possible since I went back to Korea about once or twice a year. When medical tourism was impossible, I searched for a Korean doctor here. About ten years later, I came to know American medical system better. With better knowledge and better English proficiency, I was able to receive better quality of medical care and services from American doctors. So, I tried not to see a Korean doctor anymore and changed my old family Korean doctor to an American doctor whose office was closer to my house and who had excellent reviews on google.

The medical tourism experiences of Hyun-Joo Kim, who went back to Korea to get OB/Gyn surgery in the past, were similar to Jae-Joon. Hyun-Joo had been a temporary resident for several years as she came to the United States for further study. After graduating from the university, she became a school teacher and became a permanent resident. When she was a temporary resident, she frequently went back to Korea for medical treatments, but she did not do that anymore as she became more assimilated into the US society:

> I have been in the United States about 15 years. About seven years ago, I had to have surgery, so I went back to Korea for that. At that time, I was a FOB (fresh off the boat), so I had more trust in Korean hospitals. Back then, as a temporary resident, I felt uncomfortable being hospitalized in the United States. However, I became a permanent resident, and more assimilated into the American society. So, I would not go back to Korea if I need another surgery. Now, I can handle the medical processes and procedures here. (Hyun-Joo Kim, 42, teacher, Flushing, Queens)

Old-timers commonly indicated that in addition to their greater assimilation to the US society, the increased number of Korean doctors in the NY-NJ area was another reason for their no medical tour to Korea anymore. For example, Joo-Young Park, a middle-aged entrepreneur, visited Korea for the medical purpose before. But her visits were concentrated in her early migration days:

> I had visited Korea for regular checkups and dental treatments when I first migrated to the United States in the late 1970s. Back then, there was no Korean doctor in New Jersey, which was very uncomfortable. So my husband and I often went back to Korea to see doctors. However, there are many Korean doctors in my neighborhood now, so I do not need to go back to Korea for medical care. (Joo-Young Park, 54, laundry owner, Palisades Park, New Jersey)

# *Chapter 5*

# Korean Immigrants' Medical Tourism Experience and Evaluation

## MEDICAL TOURISM EXPERIENCE

### The Arrangement of Medical Tourism

As detailed in chapter 4, social transnational ties are not only deeply associated with Korean immigrants' decision to engage in medical tourism but are also related to its arrangement. This is probably because some Korean immigrants might have difficulties in arranging medical tourism remotely while staying in the United States. More than half (61.2%) of Korean immigrant medical tourists indicated that their relatives in Korea arranged it for them. Korean residents tend to have more information about hospitals and easier access to make medical appointments. In cases in which Korean immigrants had relatives in Korea and were in frequent contact with them, their relatives made appointments for them even before they arrived in Korea. For example, Joo-Sang Yang, a 35-year-old librarian in Queens, frequently took medical tours to Korea because he regularly visited Korea to see his family and friends. He usually asked his mother to make an appointment for him before he left the United States, especially when visiting large hospitals in Korea, which usually require a longer waiting period for making arrangements than small private hospitals.

Nearly 40% of the survey respondents who have participated in medical tourism reported that they made their own medical appointments in Korea. This high proportion was possible because most Korean hospitals accept walk-in patients. Since it is easy to visit a doctor's office without an appointment in Korea, the majority of respondents who made an appointment themselves simply walked into a doctor's office when passing it on the street. Ja-Kyung Kim, a 35-year-old employee at a Korean firm in Flushing, had dental, eye, and skin treatments during her last visit to Korea. She only had to make a phone call to the dental office a few hours prior to seeing the dentist. For other treatments, she just walked into the doctors' offices, and she did not have to wait very long to receive medical treatment. Another informant, a 43-year-old housewife in Bayside, Queens, made the following comment regarding her surprise at how easy it was for her to receive a simple surgery without a prior appointment:

> Most doctors do not accept walk-ins in the United States. In contrast, in Korea, you can just go to any doctor's office without an appointment, even wearing flip-flops. Before my medical tour to Korea, I needed to have an operation to remove a sty on my eye. I did not receive the operation here and instead waited until I visited Korea. To get rid of the sty, I just walked into the eye doctor's office, and the doctor performed the operation right away. It was incredible that Korean hospitals accepted walk-ins and that they did not require appointments!

Eight respondents (5.8%) answered that their friends in Korea arranged their medical tourism. These informants, mostly young female Koreans, showed a high level of social transnational ties with their friends in Korea and a high level of interest in elective care that were popular in Korea. When they wanted to receive plastic surgery or skin treatments, they tended to ask their friends, rather than their relatives, because their peers were more familiar with the latest trends in Korea. They contacted their friends via email or Kakaotalk, a cell phone application that offers free text messages, voice calls, and video calls. Using these communication methods, they shared the medical information. Once their friends had found and recommended a doctor's office to them, the informants asked their friends to arrange their medical tours. For example, Soo-Bin Bae, a 30-year-old hairdresser, wanted to improve her physical appearance. She did not like her square-shaped chin, so she decided to have a Botox injection during her visit in Korea. Before she arrived in Korea, she had talked to her friends via Kakaotalk, and her friends in Korea had made an appointment with a famous skin doctor for her. Another female informant, Eun-Sook Jang, a 40-year-old music teacher, reported that her close friends made an appointment for her skin treatment even before she had asked them to do so. Her friends in Korea were willing to make an appointment on her behalf because they had more information and easier access to make an appointment.

Five respondents (4.1%) reported that their medical tourism was arranged through other sources, such as a Korean hospital's website. In chapter 2, I examined travel agencies' efforts to promote Korean immigrants' medical tourism and found that advertising through local Korean newspapers was their only strategy. My survey data confirms that their efforts were not very effective; only 2 of the 121 survey respondents who participated in medical tourism said that their relatives or a travel agency in the United States had arranged their medical tours to the home country. One of them, Ho-Sik Choi, a 61-year-old man who had been in the United States for more than 20 years, purchased a medical tourism package at a travel agency in New Jersey. Five years earlier, he had seen a medical tourism advertisement in a local Korean newspaper. Attracted by the low price, he called the travel agency and arranged for a physical checkup at Hanyang University Hospital, which was connected with the travel agency.

Joon-Sang Park was the other informant whose medical tourism was arranged by a travel agency. He had taken two medical tours, and the travel agency had arranged the first one. However, he did not ask the travel agency to organize his second medical tour because he had gained additional information through his first trip. People who did not use a travel agency mentioned the high commission rate as the main factor that prohibited them from purchasing a medical tourism package:

> I saw a medical tourism advertisement in the newspaper. However, I would not purchase it. The travel agency is a business that seeks economic profits. So, their medical tour package might not be as cheap as my direct contact with the hospital. Their commission rate would be high. Also, the number of hospitals affiliated with the travel agency might be limited. (Ji-Sun Han, 40, housewife, Flushing, Queens)

Korean immigrants' social networks influenced the arrangement of medical tourism as well; if their relatives or friends were medical doctors or in the medical industry, they were likely to be able to obtain more medical information or better medical services in Korea. In fact, most informants said that they were likely to know at least one medical doctor in Korea when they expanded their networks to the acquaintances of their relatives or friends. Some interviewees answered that they received advantages when their relatives, especially those who were medical doctors, arranged their medical tourism. Tae-Ho Won, an elderly Korean, regularly visited Korea for medical purposes once or twice a year, despite the fact that he had Medicare in the United States. Since he had five medical doctors among his relatives, they arranged various kinds of medical treatments for him and gave him some price and service benefits. For example, he received a discounted medical bill or even paid nothing when he saw doctors in Korea. He had no Korean naitonal health insurance, but he paid nothing when he went to see his nephew, an internal medicine doctor in Korea. His nephew also arranged other medical appointments for him to shorten his waiting time and ensure that he would receive special attention from other doctors who were his nephew's friends.

Having better social networks in Korea than in the United States also influenced the arrangement of some Korean immigrants' medical tourism. Most Korean immigrants had high educational levels and white-collar occupations prior to their migration to the United States. However, many of them experienced downward mobility in the United States. Moreover, in most cases, as an ethnic minority and as immigrants, their social networks were limited to the Korean community. Jong-Moon Kim, a university professor, emphasized that his broader social networks in Korea influenced the arrangement of his medical tourism:

> I am a university professor in the United States, but I still have narrower networks in the United States than in Korea. In Korea, I had broader networks. I even could connect with the directors of some mega hospitals, such as Yonsei Severance Hospital, through my networks in Korea. So, I would rather go back to Korea if I have a certain disease. In Korea, I had better connections that gave me opportunities to meet with better-quality doctors. When my parents arranged for my medical tourism, I had many advantages. I did not even need to wait to meet a doctor in Korea. The connections through my parents were extremely valuable. In contrast, I had to search for a physician or a hospital on Google here. In the United States, I was just "one of the patients." (Jong-Moon Kim, 42, university professor, Manhattan, New York)

## Major Cities for Medical Treatments

About two-thirds of survey respondents who participated in medical tourism (67.8%) received medical care in Seoul. There are three main reasons for their high concentration in Seoul. First, Seoul is likely to have been most Korean immigrants' hometown prior to their migration. According to the survey of Park et al. (1990), more than half of Korean immigrants reported that they had lived in Seoul before their migration to the United States, although only about a quarter of all Koreans live there. Second, about 70% of Korean immigrant medical tourists answered that they chose the city of their medical care because they had relatives in that city. Considering the high concentration of Koreans in Seoul, the capital city of the country, Korean immigrants' relatives were most likely to live in Seoul. Lastly, Seoul has more hospitals than any other city in Korea. According to a directory of hospitals made by the Korean Hospital Association (KHA), there were about 407 hospitals in Seoul, compared to 375 in Busan, 196 in Daegu, and 154 in Incheon as of August 2017. The only region with more hospitals than Seoul was Gyeonggi province, constituting the suburbs of Seoul, with 683 hospitals.

The next most commonly reported cities were Busan (9.1%), Incheon (5.8%), and Bundang (5.0%). More than 75% of Korean immigrants lived in the five largest cities in Korea prior to their migration to the United States (Park et al. 1990; Min 1996). As Busan and Incheon are the second and third largest metropolitan cities in Korea, Korean immigrants are likely to be from these cities and thus more likely to visit them than smaller cities for medical care. Also, as examined in chapter 2, the local government of Busan has actively promoted medical tourism. Bundang, a satellite city of Seoul planned and built in the early 1990s, maybe the hometown of only a small proportion of Korean immigrants, but their relatives might live there. Moreover, there are several mega hospitals in Bundang, such as SNU Hospital, Cha Medical Group, and Jesaeng Hospital.

When multiple answers were possible to choose, about two-thirds of survey respondents (71.1%) answered that they chose a particular city for their medical care because they had relatives in that city. In the previous section, I showed that more than 60% of Korean immigrants had their medical tourism arranged by their relatives. Thus, it is not surprising that the majority of them chose the city where their relatives lived as the place of their medical care. Moreover, having relatives in the city of their medical care is important because relatives can provide Korean immigrants with free accommodations. Moreover, some interviewees, especially female Koreans with young children, said that staying at a relative's house is extremely helpful for them because the relatives can also take care of their young children so that they can focus on medical treatments.

About one-third of the respondents (29.8%) chose the city they visited because it was their hometown before their migration. My informants indicated that there were two main reasons for their choice of their hometown as the city of their medical tourism: they felt more familiar with that city, and their medical records were often still stored in doctors' offices in the city after their migration to the United States, making it unnecessary for them to provide their medical history to their doctors. About one-fifth of informants chose the city because it had good hospitals. They identified several big hospitals in Seoul, such as Samsung Medical Center, Asan Medical Center and SNU Hospital, as "good hospitals." In chapter 2, I reviewed Korean local governments' various efforts to attract more Korean immigrant medical tourists. However, my survey results showed that only 2 of 121 survey respondents (1.7%) chose the city due to the promotion of medical tourism by Korean local governments.

## The Duration of Medical Tourism

I did not ask specifically about the duration of medical treatments but, rather, the total duration of their stay in Korea. Thus, most survey respondents indicated that they had stayed in Korea for a long time period. About two-thirds of them stayed in Korea for one month or longer, whereas about one-third of them stayed in Korea for less than a month. This is a longer period than I expected, because the vast majority of informants told me that it took much less time for them to receive medical care in Korea than in the United States. There seem to be three reasons for their long stay in Korea. First, as indicated in chapter 4, only 8 of 121 Korean immigrants (6.6%) answered that their visits to Korea were made only for medical reasons, while the others had multiple reasons for visiting the country, which would be likely to lengthen their stay. For example, Sang-Ho Park, a 53-year-old taxi driver, stayed in Korea for a month. He spent most of the time sightseeing with his relatives, whereas it only took several days for him to receive a checkup and dental treatments.

Second, most long-term visitors were students, housewives, or retired or unemployed individuals rather than those with jobs. Table 5.1 shows that unemployed Korean immigrants tended to stay in Korea for a longer period than their employed counterparts. Nearly half of them stayed in Korea for about a month and about one-third of them stayed in Korea for a few months or longer. On the other hand, only 14 of 69 employed Korean immigrants (20.3%) spent a few months or longer in Korea. Rather, they stayed in Korea for a much shorter time period, with nearly half staying for only a few weeks. In other words, unless they were students, housewives, retired, or unemployed, it was harder for them to take a long break because they had to work for a living in the United States.

When I interviewed the nonparticipants of medical tourism, most of them, especially the self-employed, indicated that they could not stay in Korea for a long time because of their jobs. In most cases, taking even a few days off was hard for them. In fact, four Korean informants complained that they wanted to apply for the Korean national health insurance but could not do so due to their short stay in Korea. Hye-Mi Choi, a 57-year-old entrepreneur in Queens, said that she had regularly visited Korea once every two years for medical reasons.

**Table 5.1 Duration of Stay by Employment Status**

| | *Employment Status* | | |
|---|---|---|---|
| *Duration of Stay* | *Student, Housewife, Retired, or Unemployed* | *Employed* | *All* |
| A few weeks or less | 11 (21.2%) | 30 (43.5%) | 41 (33.8%) |
| About a month | 24 (46.1%) | 25 (36.2%) | 49 (40.5%) |
| A few months or longer | 17 (32.7%) | 14 (20.3%) | 31 (25.7%) |
| Total | 52 (100.0%) | 69 (100.0%) | 121 (100.0%) |

$\chi^2$ (2, $N$ = 120) = 6.86, $p < .05$.
*Source*: Survey of 121 Korean immigrants who have participated in medical tourism to Korea.

Since she did not have health insurance in the United States, the home country was her ultimate place of medical care. However, as an entrepreneur, she could not stay in Korea for more than ten days. For this reason, she ultimately gave up receiving medical treatments in Korea. Another informant who ran a laundry in New Jersey could not stay in Korea for a long period because she needed to take care of her store, which made her hesitant to take medical tours to the home country:

> I have visited Korea about seven times since I migrated to the United States in 1997. However, I have never visited hospitals in Korea because I only visited there for one or two weeks at most. In fact, I have a myoma in my uterus, and I need surgery to get rid of it soon. Since I do not have the US health insurance, taking a medical tour to Korea is one of the options for me. However, leaving my store for a while would be a burden for me and for my family here. So, I don't know whether I should take a medical tour or not. (Hae-Lin Cho, 57, laundry owner, Palisades Park, New Jersey)

Lastly, it took at least three months for Korean immigrants to gain access to the Korean national health insurance. As indicated in Chapter 2, Korean immigrants who want to apply for the Korean national health insurance first need to receive a domestic residence card, which takes about two weeks. Then, after staying in Korea for three months, they can apply for the national health insurance with the domestic residence card. In general, medical expenses in Korea are cheaper than in the United States even without the national health insurance, but they are much cheaper with it. Thus, some Koreans, especially those who plan to receive multiple treatments or those who have severe diseases (e.g., cancer), need to stay long enough to be eligible for and receive benefits from the national health insurance program. This seemed to increase the average duration of stay among Korean immigrants who receive medical care in the home country.

## Types of Hospitals Visited for Medical Care

When multiple answers were possible to choose, about one-third of Korean immigrant medical tourists visited small private hospitals (35.5%) or university hospitals (33.1%), while about a quarter of them received medical treatments at private mega hospitals (26.5%) or dental offices (25.6%) during their stay in the home country. Fewer than 10% of them answered that they used other types of hospitals, such as public health centers or *Hanbang* offices. The primary reason for choosing these latter types of hospitals was easy accessibility due to the geographic proximity; many of them used small private hospitals or dental clinics that they could find easily near where they stayed.

On the other hand, Korean immigrants who visited university hospitals or mega private hospitals chose them for their popularity or fame. They prefer these hospitals because they are affiliated with good universities or big corporations in Korea. In fact, several interviewees told me that they visited SNU Hospital and Yonsei Severance Hospital because they considered those hospitals to be the most trustworthy due to their affiliations with the best universities. Na-Mi Kim, a 40-year-old employee at a Korean firm, said that she would go to SNU Hospital if she needed medical treatment in Korea because she believes that the doctors at SNU hospitals are the best, as the most intelligent Korean students study in the medical school at SNU.

In many cases, social network was related to the selection of the hospitals as well as the arrangements of Korean immigrants' medical tours, as discussed earlier. A few informants mentioned that they chose certain hospitals because their relatives or friends were medical doctors or staff members at those hospitals. They explained that when they knew someone at the hospital, they waited for a shorter time, paid a discounted medical bill, and received better care from the doctors and staff members. An elderly man who takes medical tours once a year told me that he went to Samsung Medical Center because his brother was a medical doctor there:

> I have been in the United States for about 30 years, and I visit Korea once a year. In fact, I have moved back and forth from Korea to the United States every six months or so. My youngest brother graduated from the medical school of Hanyang University, and now he is a doctor at Samsung Medical Center, which is one of the best hospitals in Korea. Since he was there, I chose that hospital. I paid almost nothing because he was a doctor there. Korea is more flexible than the United States in that way. (Sang-Bo Kim, 73, retired, Palisades Park, New Jersey)

Moreover, if Korean immigrants or their relatives themselves worked for the Hyundai Group, they chose Asan Medical Center because it is affiliated with the Hyundai Group. Four informants belong to this category. For example, Hae-Sung Park, a 50-year-old man who was diagnosed with a thyroid cancer in the United States, went to Asan Medical Center to get surgery. He chose that hospital not because of the doctors' ability but because of the financial benefits he received through his brother-in-law, who worked for Hyundai Engineering and Construction. The same surgery would have cost about US$20,000 in the United States, but he only paid US$300 through his brother-in-law. Another informant who had worked for Hyundai before his retirement said that he also received treatment for a discounted price at the Asan Medical Center:

> I had physical checkups twice at the Asan Medical Center when I visited Korea in the past. I had worked for the Hyundai Group for 30 years and had been a vice

president for several years. So, they offered me a huge discount for a checkup and treatments. I am not a special case—they usually give discounted prices to former executive members of the Hyundai Group. Since I had worked for the Hyundai Group for a long time, I knew the director of the hospital and received special treatment from the doctors and the staff members. (Jong-Deok Kim, 78, retired, Flushing, Queens)

## Types of Medical Care Received

The most frequent type of medical treatment among Korean immigrant medical tourists was dental care. Nearly half of them (44.6%) received dental care during their last visit to Korea. The most frequently given reason for receiving dental treatments in Korea was the lower dental costs in Korea compared to the United States. According to Ryu et al. (2015), who compared dental fees in Korea, Japan, Germany, and the United States, Korea showed much lower dental costs than the other three countries. In particular, the United States showed about 15 times higher dental costs for teeth extractions, about 18 times higher costs for amalgam fillings, and about 25 times higher costs for scaling compared to Korea.

Some Korean informants emphasized that they received the same dental treatments for much lower prices in Korea than in the United States. Jung-Hyun Doh, a 46-year-old nail salon owner, has visited Korea yearly for several years to receive dental treatments. Since her insurance does not cover dental treatments, she would have to pay US$1,000 for one amalgam filling in the United States. However, her dentists in Korea charged half the price for the same treatment and also provided dental cleanings for free. For five fillings, she would have had to pay US$5,000 in the United States. By contrast, the cost of her medical tourism was US$2,500 for five fillings and US$1,500 for the round-trip flight tickets between Seoul and New York, allowing her to save US$1,000 while also enjoying spending time with relatives and friends in Korea. Jong-Deok Kim, a 78-year-old retired man, saved even more money than Jung-Hyun, because he had eight dental implants in Korea. While his American dentist would have charged US$4,000 for one implant, his dentist in Korea charged US$1,500. Thus, by taking medical tours, he saved more than US$10,000, even after considering his airfare and other travel costs.

In addition to cheaper dental costs, some Korean immigrants believe that Korean dentists are more dexterous than American dentists due to their physical characteristics, and this belief has contributed to their choice to have dental treatments in Korea. Sang-Mi Lee, a 69-year-old woman who had been in the United States for 40 years, visited Korea to see dentists even though she had dental insurance in the United States. According to her, Korean dentists' small hands are more suitable for sophisticated dental treatments. Other interviewees also expressed similar belief in non-Korean dentists' clumsiness due to their larger hands. Anna Kim, a 27-year-old woman, stated that Korean doctors were more detailed, even for simple cleaning procedures. Hee-Jae Choi, a 58-year-old employee at a Korean firm, argued that the better dexterity of Korean dentists came from their usage of chopsticks, which are more useful than forks in training their hands for the delicate work of dentistry.

The second and third most popular medical treatments were checkups and an endoscopy or colonoscopy. About one-third of Korean immigrant medical tourists received a checkup, and about 15% of them had an endoscopy or colonoscopy during their last medical tour to the home country. They pointed out several advantages of getting these medical treatments in Korea: easier appointment procedures, the convenience of being examined in one building, and the quick turnaround time for results. A middle-aged female respondent, now an American citizen, who had taken three medical tours, explained that it was cumbersome to meet her family doctor prior to seeing a specialist. For this reason, she had an endoscopy and a colonoscopy in Korea because she liked the one-stop service at the hospitals in Korea. Another middle-aged respondent also explained that the one-stop service of Korean hospitals was a major reason that he received a checkup during his medical tours to the home country:

> In Korea, you can have one-stop service, so you can do everything once you are checked-in. You can have an endoscopy, blood test, X-ray and other examinations and treatments on the same day. In the United States, everything is specialized, so you need to visit each specialized doctor's office. If you have a stomachache, you need to go to internal medicine doctor. If you have another problem, then the doctor will refer you to another doctor. So you need to make separate appointments to see two or three doctors here. Since you have to move from one doctor's office to another, it is very inconvenient. I think the US healthcare process is too complicated, and that is the primary reason Korean immigrants, including myself, go to Korea for medical treatments. (Yong-Gyu Lim, 58, taxi driver, Bayside, Queens)

One notable finding is that Korean immigrant medical tourists received more elective care than urgent and necessary medical treatments in Korea. There were a few female respondents who had breast cancer or uterine cancer surgeries and a few male respondents who had thyroid cancer surgeries in Korea. Other than these informants, only a few received urgent or essential operations or surgeries in Korea. Regarding popular elective care, about 15% of Korean immigrants received skin treatments, and about 12.4% of them received elective eye treatments, such as LASIK or LASEK surgeries, which are used to improve one's vision rather than to cure any eye diseases. Cosmetic surgery (7.4%) was another popular form of elective care among Korean immigrants who participated in medical tours to the home country.

The types of elective care seemed to differ by gender and age. Middle-aged male Korean immigrants were more likely to receive *Hanbang* treatments, whereas the majority of respondents who received cosmetic surgery or skin treatments were young females. For them, Korean skin treatments focused more on esthetic aspects, whereas US skin treatments emphasized more therapeutic aspects. Also, these esthetic skin treatments are not covered by most US health insurance policies. Thus, Korean immigrant women who wanted to receive esthetic skin treatments preferred to go back to Korea. Jina Yoon, a 49-year-old housewife, received a laser treatment (Intense Pulsed Light, IPL) during her stay in Korea because her US insurance did not cover any esthetic skin treatments. Moreover, she felt that Korea had more advanced technologies and easier access to esthetic skin treatments. Removing a mole and getting Botox were other frequent elective skin treatments that Korean immigrants received in Korea. Regarding plastic surgery, a female informant who had a nose job and double eyelid surgeries maintained that Korea was the most advanced country for plastic surgery and that this was the main reason for her choice to receive these types of medical care there:

> I have a decent job and health insurance in the United States. I have no language barriers to access to the US healthcare because I came here when I was a high school student. However, I visited Korea seven years ago to get the nose and double-eyelid surgeries in Gangnam. Korea was the best country for me to get plastic surgery. I met many plastic surgeons in the United States, but they were not familiar with Asians' eye shapes. On the other hand, Korean plastic surgeons totally understand our eye shapes. Also, plastic surgery hospitals in Korea are very fancy. They have the most advanced technologies and the best services in the world. They even have guest rooms for the patients to stay in. I had my surgery on the 7th floor and stayed at the hotel on the 8th floor, which was very convenient for me! When I went there, there were many foreign patients from Japan, China, and Singapore. Another advantage of getting plastic surgery in Korea is that doctors are skillful because they perform hundreds of surgeries a day. Also, since there are many plastic surgery hospitals in Seoul, they offer the best services due to the excessive competition. In my case, they even offered me free mole clearing treatments because I had two major surgeries there. (Mi-Jin Noh, 34, florist, Flushing, Queens)

Approximately 12% of respondents answered that they received other types of medical treatments in Korea. In most cases, these included uterus treatments for female respondents and prostate treatments for male respondents. Interestingly, one female interviewee who had been in the United States for almost 20 years shared her experience of medical tourism for reproductive purposes:

> I tried to get pregnant for ten years after I got married. After ten years with no success, I was almost 40 years old. So, I was very anxious and worried about not being able to get pregnant. I tried artificial insemination in the United States , but that did not work. So, I visited Korea to get IVF (In Vitro Fertilization). When I did IVF for the first time, it did not work out. The second trial did not work out either, so I took my third medical tour only for the IVF. Fortunately, the third trial was successful. I then stayed in Korea for six months until I entered the second trimester, which is considered the safest period of pregnancy. When I had artificial insemination here, it cost a large amount of money even with my US health insurance. Since the IVF processes were cheaper in Korea, and since my parents were in Korea, I went to Cha Medical Group, which is famous for infertility. I am very happy with my medical tourism because I am a mother of twins now! (Ji-Yoon Choi, 46, housewife, Flushing, Queens)

## EVALUATION OF MEDICAL TOURISM

Nearly half (43.0%) of Korean immigrants who participated in medical tourism were somewhat satisfied with their experience, while the other half (56.2%) were very satisfied. The reasons for their satisfaction were similar to the reasons for their decision to engage in medical tourism as discussed in the last section of chapter 3: short waiting periods, simple medical procedures, easy communication with healthcare professionals, good services, and cheap medical costs.

However, one informant was not satisfied with his medical tourism experience and complained about it. Ji-Seok Kim, a middle-aged man who runs a business in Fort Lee, had a back surgery three years ago in Korea. He knew that the medical cost of back surgery was much lower in Korea even without Korean national health insurance. Moreover, he had a place to stay with his parents and siblings in Korea. For these reasons, he contacted a Korean hospital that specialized in back surgery and made a surgery appointment. However, he was not satisfied with the process or the results. His back did not fully recover, and his voice became husky as a side effect of the surgery. Ultimately, he bought a US health insurance policy and had another operation on his back in the United States. Fortunately, that operation went well; his back fully recovered, and his voice returned almost to normal.

Aside from this one exception, all other informants were satisfied with their medical tour experience overall, although they still reported several problems. First, like Ji-Seok, some other interviewees also pointed out the difficulty in receiving follow-up treatments. Hye-Min Cho, a middle-aged female interviewee, told me that after she had thyroid cancer surgery in Korea, her American doctor would not provide follow-up examinations and treatments for a surgery that he had not conducted. A staff member at a local travel agency also indicated that follow-up was a significant issue for some Korean immigrant medical tourists who were diagnosed with unexpected diseases during their medical tours:

> If you discover a lump in your body while doing a checkup in Korea and need treatment right away, you would have to pay extra money for a treatment that might be expensive without Korean health insurance. If you need an emergency surgery in Korea, you might have to reschedule your flight back to the United States. Also, if you have surgery in Korea, you have to fly back there for after-care. A few of my customers who bought a medical tour package learned that they had cancer or other severe diseases during their medical tours. However, when they came back to the United States with the examination results from Korea, the doctors here did not accept it. So, they had to spend extra money and time for the same examination. The majority of our customers assumed that they were healthy, so they did not consider the possibility of discovering a disease during their medical tourism. Consequently, they were embarrassed when they were diagnosed with the disease. Staying longer in Korea for further treatments or going back to Korea for follow-ups both created problems for them. (Travel agency staff member, Manhattan, New York)

Follow-up was an issue not just for Korean immigrants diagnosed with a severe disease like cancer, but also for those seeking elective care. In particular, most dental treatments needed consecutive treatments and follow-ups, so some Koreans hesitated to begin dental treatments in Korea. Jin-Hee Chang, a middle-aged woman who migrated to the United States 20 years ago was indecisive about whether or not she should start a dental implant procedure in Korea because it required follow-up treatments every six months. Two other informants also expressed indecision about starting skin treatments in Korea, because frequent follow-up treatments were needed after the first one. Sang-Hoon Baek, a 70-year-old Korean immigrant, was interested in removing spots on his face and body. However, he worried about getting proper follow-up treatments after coming back to the United States. Another female interviewee in her early 40s wanted to have an IPL in Korea, but she had decided not to do so due to the difficulty of visiting Korea regularly while her children attended schools in the United States.

In addition to the difficulty of receiving follow-up treatments, the informants disclosed concerns about the short amount of time Korean doctors spend on their patients. Regardless of their overall satisfaction with medical tourism experiences, they felt pressed for time when they received medical care in Korea. According to the informants, the doctors in Korea spent only three minutes to five minutes on them, whereas physicians in the United States spent about 20–30 minutes per visit. Jung-Soon Lee, who went back to Korea to meet a famous doctor, was shocked by how short a time the doctor spent examining her:

> After I was diagnosed with a high chance of liver cancer, I made an appointment with Dr. Kang, a liver expert at the SNU Hospital. It was very hard to make an appointment with him, so I used all of my social networks to see him. When I saw a doctor in the United States, who graduated from Harvard medical school, he spent over an hour examining me. I asked all the questions in my mind, and I discussed everything with him. However, when I met Dr. Kang in Korea, he spent just a minute with me! Dr. Kang touched my stomach twice and asked me to stand up and sit down. Then he said, "Your liver is hardened." I took a 13-hour flight to Korea to see him, but that was all I heard from him. That was it! (Jung-Soon Lee, 67, fabric designer, Manhattan, New York)

Unlike those who were only somewhat satisfied, the majority of Korean immigrant medical tourists who were very satisfied with their medical tourism experience felt that issues with follow-up treatment were not a problem for them. Yoon-A Oh, a 41-year-old woman who had had breast cancer surgery in Korea two years earlier, asked her Korean doctor to give her medical chart to her. She brought it back to the United States and showed it to her American doctor, who had no problem understanding it. She even brought a videotape that was recorded during her surgery and watched it with her American doctor. Although the doctors in the video communicated in Korean, a Korean nurse at the US hospital translated the video for her family doctor. Like Yoon-A, several interviewees argued that follow-up issues with American doctors were not a problem because the Korean hospitals provided all the necessary medical information on paper as well as on CDs.

As indicated earlier, cultural transnational ties with the home country only marginally promoted Korean immigrants' medical tourism, as only a few Koreans decided to take medical tours after seeing medical tourism advertisements in Korean newspapers. However, cultural transnational ties did help with follow-up issues. There are several Korean TV programs that specialize in health issues, and the NY-NJ-based local Korean TV stations broadcast these shows to Korean immigrants. Most Korean hospitals provided results sheets that indicated specific numeric values/levels for certain kinds of diseases for Korean immigrants, which allowed them to see whether various levels in their bodies were within normal ranges when they watched the Korean TV programs. Mi-Hee Moon described the association between cultural transnational ties and the follow-up on her medical tourism:

> When I had a checkup in Korea a year ago, the hospital gave me a booklet that indicated all the numeric values of my body. I also brought a CD that contained

> the pictures of my lung. I showed it to my family doctor in Flushing, and he understood it. Because of the paper and the CD, I had no problem getting follow-up treatments in the United States. So, I strongly encourage my friends to visit Korea for checkups because I was very satisfied with my experience. The best part was the booklet that showed all my health information. Whenever I watched a Korean TV program that indicated the normal values of a certain disease, I could compare those numbers to my numbers in the booklet. Last week, I watched a Korean health program called *Vitamin*. The MC presented the level of sodium in a normal kidney. Since I had a booklet that indicated the sodium level in my kidney, I compared that number to mine. In this way, whenever I watched the program, I could compare the figures. I love the idea of knowing the exact numbers of my body. (Mi-Hee Moon, 66, retired, Bayside, Queens)

The very satisfied Koreans also commonly indicated that an apparently trivial thing made them happy about their decision to take medical tours to the home country. For example, Joon-Ha Yoon, a 36-year-old employee in the financial industry on Wall Street, had an X-ray taken in the United States. He was shivering with a cold for half an hour while waiting for his turn, but nobody came in to check on his condition. By contrast, in Korea, a nurse provided a blanket for him while he waited for an X-ray. Seung-Ho had a similar experience. During his medical tour to Korea, he had to skip several meals for an endoscopy. He was surprised when the hospital provided a bowl of porridge for him after his endoscopy. The hospital offered porridge rather than a bowl of rice for better digestion. This bowl of porridge made him a big fan of Korean medical tourism.

Although almost all survey respondents were somewhat or very satisfied with their medical tour experience, 10.7% said that they had no future plans to visit Korea again for medical care. For most of them, their changed insurance status was one of the major contributing factors to their plans for medical tourism. Most of them had visited Korea for medical care when they were uninsured in the United States. Now that they had acquired insurance in the United States, however, they were less motivated to go back to Korea. Joo-Mi Park, a middle-aged woman who came to the United States 16 years ago, frequently returned to Korea for checkups and medical care when she did not have US health insurance. However, since becoming insured, she had not felt the need to go back to Korea for medical care:

> I had no health insurance in the US about ten years ago. So, whenever I visited Korea, I had a checkup and medical treatments, such as an endoscopy, a blood test, and a gynecological examination. I also had a hemorrhoidectomy. However, when I was diagnosed with a breast cancer five years ago, I did not go back to Korea for cancer surgery and treatment because I had US health insurance through my husband's job. Since I had all my relatives in Queens and

> had no difficulty speaking English, it was more convenient for me to get the surgery in the United States. Moreover, I did not pay much, because my insurance company covered the most of the medical bill, which was originally over US$100,000. So, I would not take medical tours to Korea anymore. (Joo-Mi Park, 43, nail salon employee, Flushing, Queens)

About one-third of respondents answered that they did not know whether they would take another medical tour to Korea. As indicated earlier, only 6.6% of Korean immigrants visited Korea only for medical purposes. Others have different purposes for their visit to Korea, such as visiting family and friends, business trips, sightseeing, and visa issues. Since they did not know when they would next visit Korea for those purposes, they also did not know whether or when they would take further medical tours to Korea.

# Conclusion

In this book, I sought to answer the following questions related to Korean immigrants' medical tours to the home country. First, how have the Korean government's policies and private sector agencies' efforts to target Korean immigrants affected their engagement with medical tourism? Second, what are Korean immigrants' coping strategies against barriers to the formal US healthcare and how are these barriers and healthcare behaviors related to their medical tours to Korea? What are the contributing factors to Korean immigrants' decisions to engage in medical tourism? Last, what are their medical tourism experiences like and how did they evaluate their medical tourism experiences? To answer the first question, I reviewed Korean governmental reports and newspaper articles published in the United States and in Korea. For the other questions, I analyzed data based on 507 surveys with Korean immigrants in the NY-NJ area, in-depth personal interviews with 100 Korean immigrants who participated in medical tourism, and in-depth personal interviews with 20 Korean immigrants who did not participate in medical tourism.

## A SUMMARY OF MAJOR FINDINGS

The development of medical tourism has begun since 2009 when the Korean government revised the medical law to legalize inviting and arranging for foreign patients. With the Korean government's and private sector agencies' efforts to attract foreign patients, the number of foreign patients who visited Korea for medical care has rapidly increased. However, their efforts were marginally influential on Korean immigrants' medical tours to the home country as less than 2% of the survey participants who had engaged in medical tourism chose the city of medical care due to the promotion by Korean local governments.

More than half of my Korean immigrant survey respondents reported that they had at least one barrier when they received healthcare in the United States. Language barriers and having no insurance were the most frequently cited barriers. Knowing these obstacles is important because they are closely related to their distinctive healthcare behaviors: preference for co-ethnic doctors, the practice of *Hanbang*, and medical tours to the home country. As expected, those who had any barrier to formal US healthcare were more likely to return to the home country for medical care. Moreover, their preference for co-ethnic physicians and use of *Hanbang* medicine in the United States were positively associated with their greater tendency to take medical tours to the home country.

I also directly asked the survey respondents who had participated in medical tourism what specific reasons led to their decision. Lower medical costs in Korea was the primary reason, followed by easier communication due to the lack of language barrier, feeling more comfortable by virtue of being in their homeland, simpler medical procedures in Korea, the better ability of Korean doctors, a shorter waiting period in Korea, and their uninsured status in the United States. Since I only asked those who actually engaged in medical tourism about the reasons for their decision, it was not possible to specify what factors contributed to decisions related to medical tourism among all Korean immigrants. Thus, I synthesized the survey data of all respondents and in-depth personal interviews regardless of whether they did or did not participate in medical tourism to examine the contributing factors to their medical tourism decision. I have found that there were three important factors to their decision: transnational social ties with the home country, health insurance status in the United States, and temporary resident status.

First and foremost, more than any other type of transnational ties, social transnational ties had the strongest positive relation to Korean immigrants' medical tours to the home country. Social transnational ties were more directly influential on medical tourism because maintaining social transnational ties had the practical benefit of providing Korean immigrants with places to stay in the home country; additionally, their social transnational ties could also help them make medical appointments there. On the contrary, cultural transnational ties and political transnational ties had less influence on medical tourism.

Second, surprisingly, my survey data indicated no significant statistical association between Korean immigrants' health insurance status and medical tourism. Their self-employment status was a mediating factor to the association between health insurance status and medical tourism. Since self-employed Korean immigrants had a lower rate of being insured than employed Koreans, I hypothesized that they would show a higher tendency to take medical tours to the home country than their counterparts. However, data did not support this expectation. To explain this unexpected finding, I speculated that long working hours and the necessity of operating a store every day may have hindered them from visiting the home country for medical care. Additionally, Korean employees of small co-ethnic businesses also had lower rates of health insurance than those who work in the general economy. Like small business owners, Koreans who work in the ethnic economy also showed a low tendency to take medical tours because they had fewer financial resources to visit the home country. Since they, along with self-employed Koreans, are more likely to be uninsured and less likely to visit the homeland for medical treatments than their counterparts in the general economy, they are marginalized from receiving medical care both in the United States and in Korea.

Lastly, temporary resident status was a strong contributing factor to Korean immigrants' medical tourism. Temporary residents were more likely to participate in medical tours to the home country because of several factors. Most of all, they are less likely to be insured and to have access to public health insurance services in the United States, such as Medicare or Medicaid, due to their temporary resident status. Moreover, temporary residents, including international students or temporary employees at Korean corporations in the United States, have stronger transnational ties with the home country and a lower level of assimilation into the American society than permanent residents or naturalized citizens.

Considering all contributing factors, Table 6.1 shows a typology of Korean immigrant medical tourists based on their health insurance status and level of social transnational ties with the home country. Although temporary resident status is another important contributing factor, it is not included in the table because it does not seem to be as influential as health insurance status or transnational ties. Moreover, as indicated earlier, it is the factor that eventually influences both the individual's health insurance status in the United States and transnational ties to the home country, the two axes in the table.

Korean immigrants with a low level of social transnational ties with the home country and with no US health insurance comprise the most marginalized group. They mostly consist of Korean small business owners and their employees. They show a low tendency to take medical tours to the home country. Rather, seeing co-ethnic doctors and receiving health services in the Korean community are their primary sources of medical care in the United States. However, due to liability issues, most Korean community organizations do not provide any major medical treatments to uninsured Koreans. Instead, several different programs provide cancer screenings, prevention programs, and other low-risk/low-liability services. Thus, when uninsured Korean immigrants with low transnational ties become ill, they are the least likely to receive proper medical care in both the United States and the home country.

**Table 6.1 Types of Korean Immigrant Medical Tourists**

| *Level of Social Transnational Ties with the Home Country* | *Health Insurance Status in the US* | |
|---|---|---|
| | *Not Insured in the US* | *Insured in the US* |
| Low | • Low tendency to take medical tours to the home country<br>• Small business owners and their employees | • Receive a checkup in the home country<br>• One-time triers |
| High | • Receive most medical care in the home country<br>• Temporary residents | • Receive elective care in the home country<br>• Professionals, big business owners, and their family members |

By contrast, if uninsured Korean immigrants have a high level of transnational ties, they will often go back to the home country, considering it as the ultimate place of medical care. They are likely to be temporary residents such as international students or resident employees. They will receive as much medical care as they can whenever they have a chance to go there. On the other hand, those who have health insurance in the United States and have a low level of transnational ties with the home country are likely to try out medical tourism just once to see what it is like. They often receive a checkup, which does not require frequent visits to the home country. Lastly, Korean immigrants who have US health insurance and maintain a high level of social transnational ties with the homeland tend to be professionals, big business owners, and their family members, and this group is likely to make frequent visits to Korea to receive elective care.

With the exception of one Korean respondent, all of the other informants expressed satisfaction with their medical tourism experiences. Yet, about one-tenth said that they would not take a medical tour again mainly because of their changed insurance status. Since they were now insured in the United States, they had fewer incentives to go back to the home country for medical care. About one-third of respondents did not know if they would take another medical tour to Korea. Since they were unsure of the next time they would visit Korea, they also did not know if or when they would take another medical tour.

## CONTRIBUTIONS AND POLICY IMPLICATIONS

### Empirical and Methodological Contributions

This book makes a significant empirical contribution to the literature on immigrant medical transnationalism by investigating Korean immigrants' medical tours to the home country with rich data sets. First, researchers have argued that each immigrant group's homogeneity or heterogeneity should be considered in health research (Arcia et al. 2001; Salant and Lauderdale 2003). In that regard, this book empirically contributes to research on ethnic health by focusing on one ethnic group in a particular area: Korean immigrants in the NY-NJ area. I practically examined how many Korean immigrants visited the home country for medical care, their reasons for medical tourism, the types of medical care they received in the home country, and their evaluation of it.

This book also contributes to the field of Asian-American studies as well as the area of minority healthcare behaviors. This book found that Korean immigrants face various barriers to formal US healthcare. Seeking medical care in the home country is one of their reactive healthcare behaviors to the barriers. Most immigration researchers have focused their research on Latino immigrants' medical tourism experiences. There are only a few studies that have examined Asian immigrants' medical tours to the home country, but they often had a small number of interviewees or had no theoretical framework. Thus, this book, which has a large sample of survey respondents and in-depth personal interviewees, in addition to a sociological framework, will make a significant contribution to the fields of Asian-American studies and Korean-American healthcare behaviors in the United States.

Second, this book methodologically contributes to the literature on immigrant medical transnationalism. Previous research on immigrants' medical tourism used mostly quantitative data with a small number of survey respondents or qualitative data with a small number of interviewees or focus group participants. Moreover, their participants or interviewees were limited to a certain age group or to those who received a particular type of medical care. Thus, this book, which has large-scale survey data with a sample of over 500 respondents and in-depth personal interviews with over 100 Korean immigrants, encompassing all ages and genders, makes a significant methodological contribution to the literature on Korean immigrants' medical tourism by utilizing both quantitative and qualitative data.

## Theoretical Contributions

This book makes a theoretical contribution to existing theories of immigrant health and immigrant transnationalism. First, it found that when Andersen's healthcare utilization model was applied, only some predisposing factors (e.g., age and educational level) were associated with Korean immigrants' medical tours to the home country. On the contrary, enabling (e.g., health insurance status) and need (e.g., current health status) factors were not significantly related to it. As expected, several immigrant factors, such as level of English proficiency and years spent in the United States, were strongly influential on Korean immigrants' medical tourism. Only a few studies have examined immigrants' coping strategies with respect to healthcare in the United States. Moreover, there is no specific framework only for Korean immigrants. Therefore, this book, which has built a framework for Korean immigrants' coping strategies, makes theoretical contributions to the literature of immigrant health.

I analyzed Korean immigrants' medical tourism as a type of medical transnationalism drawing from the transnationalism theory. As pointed out in Introduction, transnational researchers have focused on immigrants' political, economic, and social transnationalism, but have neglected medical transnationalism. While some researchers (Portes, Fernández-Kelly, and Light 2012) have given passing statements to medical transnationalism, they have not systematically examined it with empirical data. Rather, they have conceptually suggested it as one of the coping strategies for immigrants' healthcare utilization in the United States. This book has also investigated how other types of transnationalism were connected to Korean immigrants' medical transnationalism. Social transnationalism was most deeply associated with Korean immigrants' medical tourism than any other types of transnationalism. Since there was no previous study that thoroughly investigated medical transnationalism and that examined the connection between medical and other areas of transnationalism, this book will contribute to the field of immigrant transnationalism.

## Policy Implications

Major findings from this book show that Korean small business owners and employees in the ethnic economy are the most marginalized group because they have the most difficulty in getting medical care in the United States because a large proportion of them do not have health insurance. Moreover, it is difficult for them to take medical tours to the home country due to their long workdays and lack of time off. Consequently, they end up receiving inadequate medical care, both in the United States and in Korea. However, they actually have many more health problems and high stress due to the lack of leisure time caused by long work hours (Min 1990). An implication of this finding is that health programs for this marginalized group need to be initiated to help them receive appropriate and timely medical care in the host country because practically, it is almost impossible for them to visit the home country for medical care because of their obligations to their stores.

I argue that the Korean community in the United States should take the first step to making this problem more visible and developing various health programs for small business owners and their employees, including both prevention and support programs. For example, since small business owners have virtually no time to exercise outside of their stores or homes, various health prevention programs, such as a specially designed freehand exercise that they can do in their stores would be one of the preventive programs. Another possible support program is to connect this marginalized group to Korean doctors who are willing to help them and contribute to the Korean community. The vast majority of self-employed interviewees indicated that their long work hours and uninsured status prohibited them from visiting the doctor, which entails multiple processes, long hours, and a lot of money without insurance. I suggest that some of the various associations in the Korean community in the United States cooperate to build a program that connects small business owners and their employees to Korean doctors who can either visit the stores and perform regular checkups or give discounts to the uninsured.

My findings also indicate that about one-third of Korean immigrants have a language barrier to US healthcare. Easier communication with medical doctors was the major reason for their preference for co-ethnic doctors and medical tours to the home country. However, despite their language barrier, only a few informants reported that they utilized translation services at US hospitals. Those who used such services indicated that most translators were not true bilinguals. In most cases, the translators' Korean proficiency was not sufficient for communication. The lack of bilingual translators, who understand both countries' languages and cultures, became a significant structural barrier for most Korean immigrants. More support and training from health policy makers and the Korean community in the United States are needed to ensure that fluently bilingual Korean-English translators are available to facilitate the medical care of Korean immigrants.

## THE DIRECTION OF FUTURE RESEARCH

This book is only the beginning of more systematic research on immigrants' medical transnationalism. There is still much to learn about it by conducting research on several different immigrant groups to answer the following research questions. First, what are other US immigrant groups' medical tourism experiences like? As pointed out earlier, the vast majority of studies on immigrants' medical tourism have focused on Mexican immigrants, the largest immigrant group in the United States, but also a group with unique characteristics: overall, they have an extremely low rate of being insured and their home country is in very close geographical proximity to the United

States. By contrast, medical tourism experiences of other Asian immigrants have been under-researched. Therefore, it will be meaningful to explore other immigrant groups to see how different demographic, socioeconomic, health insurance status, and transnational ties affect or contribute to their medical tourism.

Second, are there any differences in medical tourism experiences between Korean immigrants in the United States and those settled in other countries? For example, several cities in the United States and Canada (e.g., New York vs. Toronto or Seattle vs. Vancouver) are similar distances from Korea but have totally different healthcare systems. Moreover, the characteristics of Korean immigrants in the United States and those in Canada may be different due to the different immigration systems of the two countries. Bearing these similarities and differences in mind, I could examine how different contributing factors and medical systems in host countries affect immigrants' decisions regarding medical tourism.

Lastly, further research could be directed at determining how healthcare systems or revised laws of both sending and receiving countries affect immigrants' medical tours to the home country. There are two possible studies regarding this. One is to see if the Patient Protection and Affordable Care Act, which is better known as Obamacare, contributed to Korean immigrants' medical tourism. I conducted most of my surveys and the in-depth personal interviews in 2013, before the enactment of Obamacare in January 2014. Since Obamacare enforces all uninsured individuals to be covered by health insurance, it would be great if I could conduct follow-up interviews with the uninsured informants after they registered for Obamacare. Then I could examine how their changed health insurance status influenced their medical tours to Korea. In fact, at the time of the interviews, some uninsured informants mentioned their interest in Obamacare and said that they would not take medical tours to Korea once they became insurance beneficiaries of Obamacare.

The findings drawn from this book indicate that Korean immigrants' medical tourism was not a simple personal decision on choosing a place of medical care. Rather, it was a complicated phenomenon influenced by various factors, such as their health insurance status, temporary resident status, various barriers to US healthcare, and transnational ties with the home country. It is my hope that my findings will serve as a foundational work in the study of immigrant transnationalism, opening a new door for the under-researched field of medical transnationalism.

*Appendix*

# Characteristics of Korean Immigrant Survey Respondents

| | $N$ | % |
|---|---|---|
| Sociodemographic Characteristics | | |
| Female | 283 | 55.8 |
| Age | | |
| 18–39 years old | 187 | 36.8 |
| 40–49 years old | 117 | 23.1 |
| 50–64 years old | 117 | 23.1 |
| 65 years old or older | 86 | 17.0 |
| Married | 331 | 65.3 |
| Educational level | | |
| Less than four-year college | 196 | 38.6 |
| 4-year college graduates | 235 | 46.4 |
| Graduate/professional school graduates | 76 | 15.0 |
| Occupational Characteristics | | |
| Type of Employer | | |
| Government/public sector/non-Korean businesses | 64 | 19.8 |
| Self-employed | 86 | 26.7 |
| Working in Korean-owned businesses | 172 | 53.5 |
| Immigrant Characteristics | | |
| Years in the United States | | |
| 1–9 years | 118 | 23.3 |
| 10–19 years | 184 | 36.3 |
| 20 years or longer | 205 | 40.4 |
| Legal status (Total $N$ = 264) | | |
| Temporary/working visa/other | 52 | 19.7 |
| Permanent residents | 84 | 31.8 |
| US citizens | 128 | 48.5 |

*(Continued)*

(*Continued*)

| | *N* | % |
|---|---|---|
| English proficiency | | |
| Not well/a little | 273 | 53.8 |
| Well/very well | 234 | 46.2 |
| Health-Related Characteristics | | |
| Current health status is good/very good | 355 | 70.0 |
| Have any health insurance | 359 | 70.8 |
| Total *N* | 507 | 100.0 |

*Note*: The total number of response for the type of employer 322, because those who were not in the labor market (e.g., retired, students, or housewives) were excluded in this question. The total number of responses for legal status is 264 because some respondents refused to indicate their legal status.
*Source*: Survey of 507 Korean immigrants in the NY-NJ area.

# Bibliography


Abraido-Lanza, A. F., Chao, M. T., & Florez, K. R. (2005). Do healthy behaviors decline with greater acculturation?: Implications for the Latino mortality paradox. *Social Science & Medicine*, *61*(6), 1243–1255.

Ahn, K. J. (2009). *South Korean transnational mothers: Familism, cultural criticism and education project*. Syracuse, NY: Syracuse University.

Akresh, I. R. (2009). Health service utilization among immigrants to the United States. *Population Research and Policy Review*, *28*(6), 795–815.

An, D. (2014). Understanding medical tourists in Korea: Cross-cultural perceptions of medical tourism among patients from the USA, Russia, Japan, and China. *Asia Pacific Journal of Tourism Research*, *19*(10), 1141–1169.

Andersen, R. (1968). *A behavioral model of families' use of health services*. Research Series No. 25. Chicago, IL: Center for Health Administration Studies, University of Chicago.

Andersen, R. M. (1995). Revisiting the behavioral model and access to medical care: Does it matter? *Journal of Health and Social Behavior*, *36*, 1–10.

Andersen, R. M., & Newman, J. F. (1973). Societal and individual determinants of medical care utilization in the United States. *The Milbank Fund Quarterly*, *51*(1), 95–124.

Arcia, E., Skinner, M., Bailey, D., & Correa, V. (2001). Models of acculturation and health behaviors among Latino immigrants to the US. *Social Science & Medicine*, *53*(1), 41–53.

Balaban, V., & Marano, C. (2010). Medical tourism research: A systematic review. *International Journal of Infectious Diseases*, *14*, e135.

Basch, L., Schiller, N. G., & Blanc, C. S. (Eds.). (1994). *Nations unbound: Transnational projects, postcolonial predicaments, and deterritorialized nation-states*. London: Psychology Press.

Bastida, E., Brown III, H. S., & Pagán, J. A. (2008). Persistent disparities in the use of health care along the US–Mexico border: An ecological perspective. *Journal Information*, *98*(11), 1987–1995.

Bergmark, R., Barr, D., & Garcia, R. (2010). Mexican immigrants in the US living far from the border may return to Mexico for health services. *Journal of Immigrant and Minority Health, 12*(4), 610–614.

Bodeker, G., & Kronenberg, F. (2002). A public health agenda for traditional, complementary, and alternative medicine. *American Journal of Public Health, 92*(10), 1582–1591.

Bookman, M. Z., & Bookman, K. R. (2007). *Medical tourism in developing countries.* New York: Palgrave Macmillan.

Boschert, S. (2007). Treating "transplant tourists" after the fact. *Internal Medicine News*. Retrieved from http://www.entrepreneur.com/tradejournals/article/print/178448629.html

Brown, H. S. (2008). Do Mexican immigrants substitute health care in Mexico for health insurance in the United States? The role of distance. *Social Science & Medicine, 67*(12), 2036–2042.

Canales, M. T., Kasiske, B. L., & Rosenberg, M. E. (2006). Transplant tourism: Outcomes of United States residents who undergo kidney transplantation overseas. *Transplantation, 82*, 1658–1661.

Carrasquillo, O., Carrasquillo, A. I., & Shea, S. (2000). Health insurance coverage of immigrants living in the United States: Differences by citizenship status and country of origin. *American Journal of Public Health, 90*(6), 917–923.

Cha, C. (2010). Health promotion and related factors among Korean goose mothers. *Asian Nursing Research, 4*(4), 205–215.

Chavez, L. R., Cornelius, W. A., & Jones, O. W. (1985). Mexican immigrants and the utilization of US health services: The case of San Diego. *Social Science & Medicine, 21*(1), 93–102.

Chin, S. Y. (1992). This, that, and the other. Managing illness in a first-generation Korean-American family. *Western Journal of Medicine, 157*(3), 305–309.

Chin, K. S., & Smith, D. (2015). A reconceptualization of state transnationalism: South Korea as an illustrative case. *Global Networks, 15*(1), 78–98.

Chinai, R., & Goswami, R. (2007). Medical visas mark growth of Indian medical tourism. *Bulletin of the World Health Organization, 85*(3), 164–165.

Choe, S. H. (2008, November 15). South Korea joins lucrative practice of inviting medical tourists to its hospitals. *The New York Times*. A15. Retrieved from http://www.nytimes.com/2008/11/16/world/asia/16medical.html

Choi, J. Y. (2013). Reconstruction of health-seeking behaviors: A comparative study of three Asian Pacific immigrant groups. *Qualitative Health Research, 23*(4), 517–530.

CNN. (2009, March). Hot destinations for medical tourism. *CNN*. Retrieved from http://www.cnn.com/2009/HEALTH/03/26/medtourism.interactive/index.html

Connell, J. (2006). Medical tourism: Sea, sun, sand and… surgery. *Tourism Management, 27*(6), 1093–1100.

Cox, C., Ma, R., Claxton, G., and Levitt, L. (2015). Analysis of 2016 premium changes and insurer participation in the ACA's health insurance marketplaces. *Report by Kaiser Family Foundation*. Retrieved from http://kff.org/health-reform/issue-brief/analysis-of-2016-premium-changes-and-insurer-participation-in-the-affordable-care-acts-health-insurance-marketplaces/.

Dawn, S. K., & Pal, S. (2011). Medical tourism in India: Issues, opportunities and designing strategies for growth and development. *International Journal of Multidisciplinary Research*, *1*(3), 7–10.

De Arellano, A. B. R. (2007). Patients without borders: The emergence of medical tourism. *International Journal of Health Services*, *37*(1), 193–198.

De Gagne, J. C., Oh, J., So, A., & Kim, S. S. (2014). The healthcare experiences of Koreans living in North Carolina: A mixed methods study. *Health & Social Care in the Community*, *22*(4), 417–428.

Derose, K. P., Escarce, J. J., & Lurie, N. (2007). Immigrants and health care: Sources of vulnerability. *Health Affairs*, *26*(5), 1258–1268.

Derose, K. P., Bahney, B. W., Lurie, N., & Escarce, J. J. (2009). Immigrants and health care access, quality, and cost. *Medical Care Research and Review*, *66*(4), 355–408.

Ell, Kathleen & Irma Castaneda. (1998). Health care seeking behavior. In Sana Loue (Ed.) *Handbook of Immigrant Health*. Berlin: Springer Science & Business Media.

Faist, T. (2000). Transnationalization in international migration: Implications for the study of citizenship and culture. *Ethnic and Racial Studies*, *23*(2), 189–222.

Ferguson, W. J., & Candib, L. M. (2002). Culture, language, and the doctor-patient relationship. *FMCH Publications and Presentations*, *61*, 353–361.

Fetscherin, M., & Stephano, R. M. (2016). The medical tourism index: Scale development and validation. *Tourism Management*, *52*, 539–556.

Fisher, C., & Sood, K. (2014). What is driving the growth in medical tourism? *Health Marketing Quarterly*, *31*(3), 246–262.

Flores, G. (2000). Culture and the patient-physician relationship: Achieving cultural competency in health care. *The Journal of Pediatrics*, *136*(1), 14–23.

Foner, N. (1997). What's new about transnationalism?: New York immigrants today and at the turn of the century. *Diaspora: A Journal of Transnational Studies*, *6*(3), 355–375.

Fong, V. L. (2008). The other side of the healthy immigrant paradox: Chinese sojourners in Ireland and Britain who return to China due to personal and familial health crises. *Culture, Medicine, and Psychiatry*, *32*(4), 627–641.

Gahlinger, P. (2008). *The medical tourism travel guide: Your complete reference to top-quality, low-cost dental, cosmetic, medical care & surgery overseas*. North Branch, MN: Sunrise River Press.

Ganguli, S., & Ebrahim, A. H. (2017). A qualitative analysis of Singapore's medical tourism competitiveness. *Tourism Management Perspectives*, *21*, 74–84.

Garcia-Altes, A. (2005). The development of health tourism services. *Annals of Tourism Research*, *32*(1), 262–266.

Gorman, B. K., Read, J. N. G., & Krueger, P. M. (2010). Gender, acculturation, and health among Mexican Americans. *Journal of Health and Social Behavior*, *51*(4), 440–457.

Gray, B., & Stoddard, J. J. (1997). Patient-physician pairing: Does racial and ethnic congruity influence selection of a regular physician? *Journal of Community Health*, *22*(4), 247–259.

Green, S. T. (2008). Medical tourism – a potential growth factor in infection medicine and public health. *Journal of Infection*, *57*(5), 429.

Guarnizo, L. E., & Smith, M. P. (1998). The locations of transnationalism. *Transnationalism from Below*, *6*, 3–34.

Han, G. S. (1997). The rise of western medicine and revival of traditional medicine in Korea: A brief history. *Korean Studies*, *21*, 96–121.

Han, G. S. (2000). Traditional herbal medicine in the Korean community in Australia: A strategy to cope with health demands of immigrant life. *Health*, *4*(4), 426–454.

Han, G. S. (2001). The provision of *Hanbang* herbal medicine in the Korean community in Australia: Entrepreneurial or caring for fellow Koreans? *Australian Health Review*, *24*(4), 146–155.

Han, H., & Hyun, S. S. (2014). Medical hotel in the growth of global medical tourism. *Journal of Travel & Tourism Marketing*, *31*(3), 366–380.

Han, H., & Hyun, S. S. (2015). Customer retention in the medical tourism industry: Impact of quality, satisfaction, trust, and price reasonableness. *Tourism Management*, *46*, 20–29.

Harryono, M., Huang, Y. F., Miyazawa, K., & Sethaput, V. (2006). Thailand medical tourism cluster. *Harvard Business School Microeconomics of Competitiveness*, 1–31.

Hill, L., Hofstetter, C. R., Hovell, M., Lee, J., Irvin, V., & Zakarian, J. (2006). Koreans' use of medical services in Seoul, Korea and California. *Journal of Immigrant and Minority Health*, *8*(3), 273–280.

Hoefer, M., Rytina, N., & Baker B. C. (2009). *Estimates of the unauthorized immigrant population residing in the United States: January 2009*. Office of Homeland Security.

Homedes, N., & LaBrec, P. (1991). Health services utilization across the Arizona-Sonora Border: A binational maternal and child health project. Southwest Border Rural Health Research Center, College of Medicine, University of Arizona. Monograph, (28).

Horowitz, M. D., Rosensweig, J. A., & Jones, C. A. (2007). Medical tourism: Globalization of the healthcare marketplace. *Medscape General Medicine*, *9*(4), 33–44.

Horton, S., & Cole, S. (2011). Medical returns: Seeking health care in Mexico. *Social Science & Medicine*, *72*(11), 1846–1852.

Hsiao, A. F., Wong, M. D., Goldstein, M. S., Yu, H. J., Andersen, R. M., Brown, E. R., Becerra, L. M., & Wenger, N. S. (2006). Variation in complementary and alternative medicine (CAM) use across racial/ethnic groups and the development of ethnic-specific measures of CAM use. *Journal of Alternative & Complementary Medicine*, *12*(3), 281–290.

Hu, D. J., & Covell, R. M. (1986). Health care usage by Hispanic outpatients as a function of primary language. *Western Journal of Medicine*, *144*(4), 490–493.

Hurh, W. M., & Kim, K. C. (1990). Correlates of Korean immigrants' mental health. *The Journal of Nervous and Mental Disease*, *178*(11), 703–711.

International Medical Travel Journal. (2013, March 15). *Singapore Medical Tourism Is Recovering*. Retrieved from https://www.imtj.com/news/singapore-medical-tourism-recovering/

Itzigsohn, J., Cabral, C. D., Medina, E. H., & Vazquez, O. (1999). Mapping Dominican transnationalism: Narrow and broad transnational practices. *Ethnic and Racial Studies*, *22*(2), 316–339.

Itzigsohn, J. (2000). Immigration and the boundaries of citizenship: The institutions of immigrants' political transnationalism. *International Migration Review*, 1126–1154.

Jang, Y., Kim, G., & Chiriboga, D. A. (2005). Health, healthcare utilization, and satisfaction with service: Barriers and facilitators for older Korean Americans. *Journal of the American Geriatrics Society*, *53*(9), 1613–1617.

Jenkins, C. N., Le, T., McPhee, S. J., Stewart, S., & Ha, N. T. (1996). Health care access and preventive care among Vietnamese immigrants: Do traditional beliefs and practices pose barriers? *Social Science & Medicine*, *43*(7), 1049–1056.

Jeong, Y. J., You, H. K., & Kwon, Y. I. (2013). One family in two countries: Mothers in Korean transnational families. *Ethnic and Racial Studies*, (ahead-of-print), 1–19.

Jun, J., & Oh, K. M. (2015). Framing risks and benefits of medical tourism: A content analysis of medical tourism coverage in Korean American community newspapers. *Journal of Health Communication*, *20*(6), 720–727.

Juon, H. S., Choi, Y., & Kim, M. T. (2000). Cancer screening behaviors among Korean-American women. *Cancer Detection and Prevention*, *24*(6), 589–601.

Kamimura, A., Christensen, N., Tabler, J., Ashby, J., & Olson, L. M. (2013). Patients utilizing a free clinic: Physical and mental health, health literacy, and social support. *Journal of Community Health*, *38*(4), 716–723.

Kang, Y. (2012). Transnational motherhood in the making of global kids: South Korean educational migrants in Singapore. In C. Pluss, & K. Chan (Eds.), *Living intersections: Transnational migrant identifications in Asia* (pp. 149–166). Dordrecht: Springer Netherlands.

Kasinitz, P., Waters, M. C., Mollenkopf, J. H., & Anil, M. (2002). Transnationalism and the children of immigrants in contemporary New York. In P. Levitt, & M. C. Waters (Eds.) *The changing face of home: The transnational lives of the second generation*, (pp. 96–122). New York: Russell Sage Foundation.

Keckley, P. H., & Underwood, H. R. (2008). Medical tourism: Consumers in search of value. *Deloitte Center for Health Solutions*. Retrieved from http://www.deloitte.com/assets/Dcom-unitedStates/Local%20Assets/Documents/us_chs_MedicalTourismStudy(3).pdf

Kim, I. (1981). *New urban immigrants: The Korean community in New York*. Princeton: Princeton University Press.

Kim, M., Han, H. R., Kim, K. B., & Duong, D. N. (2002). The use of traditional and Western medicine among Korean American elderly. *Journal of Community Health*, *27*(2), 109–120.

Kim, J., & Chan, M. M. (2004). Factors influencing preferences for alternative medicine by Korean Americans. *The American Journal of Chinese Medicine*, *32*(2), 321–329.

Kim, K. (2009). Change and challenge of Korean family in the era of globalization: Centering transnational families. *Journal of Ritsumeikan Social Sciences and Humanities*, *1*, 167–187.

Kim, G., Aguado Loi, C. X., Chiriboga, D. A., Jang, Y., Parmelee, P., & Allen, R. S. (2011). Limited English proficiency as a barrier to mental health service use: A study of Latino and Asian immigrants with psychiatric disorders. *Journal of Psychiatric Research*, *45*(1), 104–110.

Kim, S., Lee, J., & Jung, J. (2013). Assessment of medical tourism development in Korea for the achievement of competitive advantages. *Asia Pacific Journal of Tourism Research, 18*(5), 421–445.

Kivisto, P. (2003). Social spaces, transnational immigrant communities, and the politics of incorporation. *Ethnicities, 3*(1), 5–28.

Ko, T. (2011). Medical tourism system model. *International Journal of Tourism Sciences, 11*(1), 17–51.

Ko, L. K., Taylor, V. M., Yoon, J., Copeland, W. K., Hwang, J. H., Lee, E. J., & Inadomi, J. (2016). The impact of medical tourism on colorectal screening among Korean Americans: A community-based cross-sectional study. *BMC Cancer, 16*(1), 931.

Koechlin, F., Lorenzoni, L., & Schreyer, P. (2010). Comparing price levels of hospital services across countries. *OECD Health Working Papers*. Retrieved from http://www.oecd-ilibrary.org/docserver/download/5km91p4f3rzw.pdf?expires=1425454467&id=id&accname=guest&checksum=16B226A3B41D2BF133437CF8E2F57982

Kraut, A. M. (1990). Healers and strangers: Immigrant attitudes toward the physician in America—A relationship in historical perspective. *JAMA, 263*(13), 1807–1811.

Kronenberg, F., Cushman, L. F., Wade, C. M., Kalmuss, D., & Chao, M. T. (2006). Race/ethnicity and women's use of complementary and alternative medicine in the United States: Results of a national survey. *American Journal of Public Health, 96*(7), 1236–1242.

Kung, W. W. (2004). Cultural and practical barriers to seeking mental health treatment for Chinese Americans. *Journal of Community Psychology, 32*(1), 27–43.

Kwak, M. J., & Hiebert, D. (2010). Globalizing Canadian education from below: A case study of transnational immigrant entrepreneurship between Seoul, Korea and Vancouver Canada. *Journal of International Migration and Integration, 11*(2), 131–153.

Kwong, Peter. (1997). *Forbidden workers: Illegal Chinese immigrants and American labor*. New York: Free Press.

Landeck, M., & Garza, C. (2003). Utilization of physician health care services in Mexico by US Hispanic border residents. *Health Marketing Quarterly, 20*(1), 3–16.

LaVeist, T. A., & Nuru-Jeter, A. (2002). Is doctor-patient race concordance associated with greater satisfaction with care? *Journal of Health and Social Behavior, 43*(September), 296–306.

LaVeist, T. A., Nuru-Jeter, A., & Jones, K. E. (2003). The association of doctor-patient race concordance with health services utilization. *Journal of Public Health Policy, 24*(3), 312–323.

Leclere, F. B., Jensen, L., & Biddlecom, A. E. (1994). Health care utilization, family context, and adaptation among immigrants to the United States. *Journal of Health and Social Behavior, 35*(4), 370–384.

Lee, J. Y., Kearns, R. A., & Friesen, W. (2010). Seeking affective health care: Korean immigrants' use of homeland medical services. *Health & Place, 16*(1), 108–115.

Lee, H. (2010). "I am a Kirogi Mother": Education exodus and life transformation among Korean transnational women. *Journal of Language, Identity, and Education, 9*(4), 250–264.

Lee, J. H., & Park, N. R. (2013). MICE and Medical Tourism in Singapore. Korea Institute for International Economic Policy (KIEP) Research Paper. World Economic Update, 13–49.

Lee, H., Wright, K. B., O'Connor, M., & Wombacher, K. (2014). Framing medical tourism: An analysis of persuasive appeals, risks and benefits, and new media features of medical tourism broker websites. *Health Communication*, *29*(7), 637–645.

Levitt, P. (2001). Transnational migration: Taking stock and future directions. *Global Networks*, *1*(3), 195–216.

Levitt, P., & Waters, M. C. (Eds.). (2002). *The changing face of home: The transnational lives of the second generation*. New York: Russell Sage Foundation.

Levitt, P., DeWind, J., & Vertovec, S. (2003). International perspectives on transnational migration: An introduction. *International Migration Review*, *37*(3), 565–575.

Lunt, N., & Carrera, P. (2010). Medical tourism: Assessing the evidence on treatment abroad. *Maturitas*, *66*(1), 27–32.

Ma, G. X. (1999). Between two worlds: The use of traditional and Western health services by Chinese immigrants. *Journal of Community Health*, *24*(6), 421–437.

Macias, E. P., & Morales, L. S. (2001). Crossing the border for health care. *Journal of Health Care for the Poor and Underserved*, *12*(1), 77–87.

MacReady, N. (2007). Developing countries court medical tourists. *Lancet*, *369*(9576), 1849–1850.

Mary, S. R. (2014). Medical tourism in Asia—An overview. *IRMJCR*, *10*, 122–137.

Mattoo, A., & Rathindran, R. (2006). How health insurance inhibits trade in health care. *Health Affairs*, *25*(2), 358–368.

McAlister, E. (1998). The Madonna of 115th street revisited: Vodou and Haitian Catholicism in the age of transnationalism. In R. S. Warner, & J. G. Wittner (Eds.), *Gatherings in diaspora: Religious communities and the new immigration* (pp. 123–160). Philadelphia: Temple University Press.

Messias, D. K. H. (2002). Transnational health resources, practices, and perspectives: Brazilian immigrant women's narratives. *Journal of Immigrant Health*, *4*(4), 183–200.

Miller, J. K. (1990). Use of traditional Korean health care by Korean immigrants to the United States. *Sociology and Social Research*, *75*, 38–43.

Milstein, A., & Smith, M. (2006). America's new refugees-seeking affordable surgery offshore. *New England Journal of Medicine*, *355*(16), 1637–1640.

Min, P. G. (1984). From white-collar occupations to small business: Korean immigrants' occupational adjustment. *The Sociological Quarterly*, *25*(3), 333–352.

Min, P. G. (1990). Problems of Korean immigrant entrepreneurs. *International Migration Review*, *24*(3), 436–455.

Min, P. G. (1991). Cultural and economic boundaries of Korean ethnicity: A comparative analysis. *Ethnic and Racial Studies*, *14*(2), 225–241.

Min, P. G. (1992). The structure and social functions of Korean immigrant churches in the United States. *International Migration Review*, *26*, 1370–1394.

Min, P. G. (1996). *Caught in the middle: Korean communities in New York and Los Angeles*. Berkeley: University of California Press.

Mm, P. G. (2001). Koreans: An "Institutionally Complete Community" in New York. In N. Foner (Ed.), *New Immigrants in New York* (pp. 173–200). New York: Columbia University Press.

Min, P. G., & Bozorgmehr, M. (2003). United States: The entrepreneurial cutting edge. In R. Kloosterman, & J. Rath (Eds.), *Immigrant Entrepreneurs: Venturing Abroad in the Age of Globalization* (pp. 17–37). Oxford: Berg.

Min, P. G. (Ed.). (2005). *Asian Americans: Contemporary trends and issues*. Thousand Oaks, CA: Sage Publications.

Min, P. G. (2008). *Ethnic solidarity for economic survival: Korean greengrocers in New York City*. New York: Russell Sage Foundation Publications.

Min, P. (2010). *Preserving ethnicity through religion in America: Korean Protestants and Indian Hindus across generations*. New York: NYU Press.

Min, P. G. (2012a). Population growth and racial composition in Korean enclaves in the New York-New Jersey Area, 1980–2010. Research Report 5, The Research Center for Korean Community at Queens College.

Min, P. G. (2012b). Transnational cultural activities among Korean immigrants in the New York-New Jersey Area: A content analysis. *Journal Studies of Koreans Abroad*, *28*, 49–83.

Min, P. G. (2013). *Koreans in North America: Their Experiences in the Twenty-First Century*. Lanhanm, MD: Lexington Books.

Min, P. G., & Jang, S. H. (2015). The diversity of Asian immigrants' participation in religious institutions in the United States. *Sociology of Religion*, *76*(3), 253–274.

Moghavvemi, S., Ormond, M., Musa, G., Isa, C. R. M., Thirumoorthi, T., Mustapha, M. Z. B., & Chandy, J. J. C. (2017). Connecting with prospective medical tourists online: A cross-sectional analysis of private hospital websites promoting medical tourism in India, Malaysia, and Thailand. *Tourism Management*, *58*, 154–163.

Noh, S., Kwak, M. J., & Han, J. J. H. (2013). Transnational interactions among Korean immigrants in Toronto: Family ties and socioeconomic, cultural, and political participation. *Koreans in North America: Their Experiences in the Twenty-First Century*, 121–134.

Noree, T., Hanefeld, J., & Smith, R. (2016). Medical tourism in Thailand: A cross-sectional study. *Bulletin of the World Health Organization*, *94*(1), 30–36.

OECD. (2011). Medical tourism: treatments, markets, and health system implications: A scoping review. *Directorate for Employment, Labour and Social Affairs*. Retrieved from http://www.oecd.org/els/health-systems/48723982.pdf

Oh, S. H. (2007). *Immigrant communities and ethnic linkages: Suburban Koreans in the New York-New Jersey Metropolitan Area*. Retrieved from ProQuest Digital Dissertations.

Oh, K. M., Jun, J., Zhou, Q., & Kreps, G. (2014). Korean American women's perceptions about physical examinations and cancer screening services offered in Korea: The influences of medical tourism on Korean Americans. *Journal of Community Health*, *39*(2), 221–229.

Okie, S. (2007). Immigrants and health care—at the intersection of two broken systems. *New England Journal of Medicine*, *357*(6), 525–529.

Ormond, M., Mun, W. K., & Khoon, C. C. (2014). Medical tourism in Malaysia: How can we better identify and manage its advantages and disadvantages? *Global Health Action*, *7*(1), 25201.

Pang, K. Y. (1991). *Korean elderly women in America: Everyday life, health, and illness*. New York: AMS Press, Inc.

Park, I. S. H., Fawcett, J., Arnold, F., & Gardner, R. (1990). Korean immigrants to the United States: A pre-departure analysis. *Papers of the East-West Population Institute*, no. 114. Hawaii: Population Institute, East-West Center.

Portes, A., Guarnizo, L. E., & Landolt, P. (1999). The study of transnationalism: Pitfalls and promise of an emergent research field. *Ethnic and Racial Studies*, *22*(2), 217–237.

Portes, A. (2001). Introduction: The debates and significance of immigrant transnationalism. *Global Networks*, *1*(3), 181–194.

Portes, A. (2003). Conclusion: Theoretical convergencies and empirical evidence in the study of immigrant transnationalism. *International Migration Review*, 37(3), 874–892.

Portes, A., Fernández-Kelly, P., & Light, D. (2012). Life on the edge: Immigrants confront the American health system. *Ethnic and Racial Studies*, *35*(1), 3–22.

Pourat N., Lubben J., Wallace S. P., Moon A. (1999). Predictors of use of traditional Korean healers among elderly Koreans in Los Angeles. *Gerontologist*, *39*, 711–719.

Reddy, S. G., York, V. K., & Brannon, L. A. (2010). Travel for treatment: Students' perspective on medical tourism. *International Journal of Tourism Research*, *12*(5), 510–522.

Reed, C. M. (2008). Medical tourism. *Medical Clinics of North America*, *92*(6), 1433–1446.

Ryu, H., Young, W. B., & Park, C. (2001). Korean American health insurance and health services utilization. *Research in Nursing & Health*, *24*(6), 494–505.

Saha, S., Komaromy, M., Koepsell, T. D., & Bindman, A. B. (1999). Patient-physician racial concordance and the perceived quality and use of health care. *Archives of Internal Medicine*, *159*(9), 997–1004.

Salant, T., & Lauderdale, D. S. (2003). Measuring culture: A critical review of acculturation and health in Asian immigrant populations. *Social Science & Medicine*, *57*(1), 71–90.

Schiller, N. G., Basch, L., & Blanc Szanton, C. (1992). Transnationalism: A new analytic framework for understanding migration. *Annals of the New York Academy of Sciences*, *645*(1), 1–24.

Shin, J. K. (2002). Help-seeking behaviors by Korean immigrants for depression. *Issues in Mental Health Nursing*, *23*(5), 461–476.

Shin, H., Song, H., Kim, J., & Probst, J. C. (2005). Insurance, acculturation, and health service utilization among Korean-Americans. *Journal of Immigrant Health*, *7*(2), 65–74.

Smith, M. P., & Guarnizo, L. E. (Eds.). (1998). *Transnationalism from below*. New Brunswick: Transaction Books.

Smith, R. (2005). *Mexican New York: Transnational lives of new immigrants*. California: University of California Press.

Sohn, L., & Harada, N. D. (2004). Time since immigration and health services utilization of Korean-American older adults living in Los Angeles County. *Journal of the American Geriatrics Society*, *52*(11), 1946–1950.

Son, J. (2013). Assimilation and health service utilization of Korean immigrant women. *Qualitative Health Research*, *23*(11), 1528–1540.

Song, Y. J. (2009). The South Korean health care system. *JMAJ*, *52*(3), 206–209.

Song, J. (2010). Language ideology and identity in transnational space: Globalization, migration, and bilingualism among Korean families in the USA. *International Journal of Bilingual Education and Bilingualism*, *13*(1), 23–42.

Song, H. J., Han, H. R., Lee, J. E., Kim, J. Y., Kim, K. B., Ryu, J. P., & Kim, M. (2010). Does access to care still affect health care utilization by immigrants? Testing of an empirical explanatory model of health care utilization by Korean American immigrants with high blood pressure. *Journal of Immigrant and Minority Health*, *12*(4), 513–519.

Song, J. (2012). The struggle over class, identity, and language: A case study of South Korean transnational families. *Journal of Sociolinguistics*, *16*(2), 201–217.

Sultana, S., Haque, A., Momen, A., & Yasmin, F. (2014). Factors affecting the attractiveness of medical tourism destination: An empirical study on India-Review Article. *Iranian Journal of Public Health*, *43*(7), 867.

Tang, C. F., & Lau, E. (2017). Modelling the demand for inbound medical tourism: The case of Malaysia. *International Journal of Tourism Research*, *19*(5), 584–593.

Takada, E., Ford, J. M., & Lloyd, L. S. (1998). Asian Pacific Islander Health. In S. Loue (Ed.), *Handbook of Immigrant Health*, 303–327. New York: Plenum.

Tawichai, T. & Antaseeda, P. (2002, June 3). Thai medicine takes on the world. *Bangkok Post*, 3.

Teh, I. (2007). Healthcare tourism in Thailand: Pain ahead? *Asia-Pacific Biotech News*, *11*(8), 493–497.

Terzi, E., Kern, T. & Kohnen, T. (2008). Complications after refractive surgery abroad. *Ophthalmologe*, *105*, 474–479.

Thompson, W. W. (1993). Cross-border health care utilization and practices of Mexican-Americans in the Lower Rio Grande Valley. *Border Health Journal*, *9*(2), 1–9.

US Department of Commerce. (2005). Office of Travel and Tourism Industries Survey of International Air Travelers US to Overseas and Mexico by Birth and Citizenship. 2004 report.

Viruell-Fuentes, E. A. (2007). Beyond acculturation: Immigration, discrimination, and health research among Mexicans in the United States. *Social Science & Medicine*, *65*(7), 1524–1535.

Waldinger, R., & Fitzgerald, D. (2004). Transnationalism in question. *American Journal of Sociology*, *109*(5), 1177–1195.

Wallace, S. P., Mendez-Luck, C., & Castañeda, X. (2009). Heading south: Why Mexican immigrants in California seek health services in Mexico. *Medical Care*, *47*(6), 662–669.

Wang, L. (2007). Immigration, ethnicity, and accessibility to culturally diverse family physicians. *Health & Place*, *13*(3), 656–671.

Wang, L., Rosenberg, M., & Lo, L. (2008). Ethnicity and utilization of family physicians: A case study of Mainland Chinese immigrants in Toronto, Canada. *Social Science & Medicine*, *67*(9), 1410–1422.

Wang, L., & Kwak, M. J. (2015). Immigration, barriers to healthcare and transnational ties: A case study of South Korean immigrants in Toronto, Canada. *Social Science & Medicine*, *133*, 340–348.

Wong, K. M., Velasamy, P., & Arshad, T. N. T. (2014). Medical tourism destination SWOT analysis: A case study of Malaysia, Thailand, Singapore, and India. In *SHS Web of Conferences* (Vol. 12, 01037). EDP Sciences.

Wu, A. P., Burke, A., & LeBaron, S. (2007). Use of traditional medicine by immigrant Chinese patients. *Family Medicine-Kansas City*, *39*(3), 195–200.

Wu, M. C., Kviz, F. J., & Miller, A. M. (2009). Identifying individual and contextual barriers to seeking mental health services among Korean American immigrant women. *Issues in Mental Health Nursing*, *30*(2), 78–85.

Xing, H. (1998). International trade in Health Services. A Development Perspective. The Case of China. *UNCTAD-WHO Joint Publication*. [Doc. Symbol: UNCTAD/ITCD/TSB/5-WHO/TFHE/98.1].

Yang, P. Q. (2006). Transnationalism as a new mode of immigrant labor market incorporation: Preliminary evidence from Chinese transnational migrants. *Journal of Chinese Overseas*, *20*(2), 173–192.

Yoo, H. C., Gee, G. C., & Takeuchi, D. (2009). Discrimination and health among Asian American immigrants: Disentangling racial from language discrimination. *Social Science & Medicine*, *68*(4), 726–732.

Yoon, I. J. (1991). The changing significance of ethnic and class resources in immigrant businesses: The case of Korean immigrant businesses in Chicago. *International Migration Review*, *25*(2), 303–332.

Zhang, J., & Verhoef, M. J. (2002). Illness management strategies among Chinese immigrants living with arthritis. *Social Science & Medicine*, *55*(10), 1795–1802.

## KOREAN BIBLIOGRAPHY

Ahn, H. L., Kim, E. H., & Hurh, J. (2009, May 12). '동포 입소문' 외국 환자 유치 도움. *Joongang Ilbo*. Retrieved from http://article.joins.com/news/article/article.asp?total_id=3603768.

Ahn, H. L., & Hurh, J. (2009, May 12). 한국 390만—미국 3000만원 … 동포들 '건강 검진' 몰려온다. *Joongang Ilbo*. Retrieved from http://article.joins.com/news/article/article.asp?total_id=3603799&cloc=olink|article|default.

Bae, J. Y. (2012). 1건당 40~50% 수수료… 쌍커풀 수술 1000만원 들기도. *Joongang Ilbo*, 18 November. Retrieved from http://article.joins.com/news/article/article.asp?total_id=9916188&cloc=joongang%7Carticle%7Crelated_news.

Byun, H. W. (2009, February 18). "외국인 환자 모셔라" 강남구·병원 손잡았다. *Chosun Ilbo*. Retrieved from http://news.chosun.com/site/data/html_dir/2009/02/18/2009021800017.html.

Choi, S. T. (2010a, January 20). 작년 한인 관광사 이용 고객 분석해보니…하와이 줄고 크루즈 늘고. *Koreadaily*. Retrieved from http://m.koreadaily.com/read.asp?art_id=974632.

Choi, H. S. (2010b, January 14). 한국병원 진료 상담해 드립니다…SK 컨설팅, 의료관광 포털 상반기 개설. *Koreadaily*. Retrieved from http://www.koreadaily.com/news/read.asp?art_id=971614.

Choi, S. T. (2010c, December 21). 한국의료관광 한인들 '암검사' 가장 중점. *Koreadaily*. Retrieved from http://www.koreadaily.com/news/read.asp?art_id=1131751.

Choi, M. J. (2012, August 16). 2013 전문대 신설 이색학과. *Chosun Ilbo*. Retrieved from http://news.chosun.com/site/data/html_dir/2012/08/15/2012081500905.html.

Chung, D. Y. (2011a, April 5). 미국 의료보험으로 한국서 검진·진료. *The Korea Times*. Retrieved from http://sf.koreatimes.com/article/653836.

Chung, B. S. (2011b, July 2). 일본 여성들도 원정출산 오는 이 병원. *Chosun Ilbo*. Retrieved from http://news.chosun.com/site/data/html_dir/2011/07/01/2011070101071.html.

Hurh, M. K., Cho, H. S., Choi, Y. G., Park, H. J., & Chung, K. T. (2013). The Analysis of International Competitiveness and Policy Objects of Medical Tourism. Issue Paper Institute for Industrial Economics and Trade (KIET).

Jin, S. C. (2011, May 27). '한국 의료관광' 미국인들 폭발적으로 늘었다. *Koreadaily*. Retrieved from http://www.koreadaily.com/news/read.asp?art_id=1204058.

Kang, G. H. (2013, August 28). Feel Gangnam style at Girls Generation's favorite restaurant. *Joongang Ilbo*. Retrieved from http://news.joins.com/article/12452328.

KHIDI (Korea Health Industry Development Institute). (2010). Statistics on International Patients in Korea. Report, Korea Health Industry Development Institute (KHIDI), Korea.

KHIDI. (2013). 외국인환자통계. Statistics on International Patients in Korea. Report, Korea Health Industry Development Institute (KHIDI), Korea.

KHIDI. (2016). Statistics on International Patients in Korea. Report, Korea Health Industry Development Institute (KHIDI), Korea.

Kim, E. H. (2009, April 27). Korean doctors are traveling abroad to attract foreign patients. *Joongang Ilbo*. Retrieved from http://article.joins.com/news/article/article.asp?total_id=3585659.

Kim, C. J. (2011, December 29). 우리 의술 우습게 봐? 오기로 뛰었죠. *Chosun Ilbo*. Retrieved from http://news.chosun.com/site/data/html_dir/2011/12/29/2011122900001.html.

Kim, C. R., & Kang, M. S. (2012, February 18). 쌍꺼풀수술 한국인은 80만원, 중국인엔 250만원 받더라. *Chosun Ilbo*. Retrieved from http://news.chosun.com/site/data/html_dir/2012/02/17/2012021701296.html.

Kim, H. J., & Ham, J. H. (2012, August 10). 고국 의료관광' 맹신 금물. *Koreadaily*. Retrieved from http://dc.koreatimes.com/article/745490.

Ko, J. K. (2010, October 29). Sheena Easton, Peter Fonda, and other Hollywood stars are coming. *Joongang Ilbo*. Retrieved from http://gangnam.joins.com/news/article/Article.aspx?total_id=4581087&sc=&mc=.

KOTRA. (2009). 미국인들, 저렴한 의료서비스 찾아 아시아로 몰려든다. Retrieved from http://www.globalwindow.org/gw/overmarket/GWOMAL020M.html?BBS_ID=10&MENU_CD=M10103&UPPER_MENU_CD=M10102&MENU_STEP=3&ARTICLE_ID=2100004.

KOTRA (Korea Trade Investment Promotion Agency). (2011). 미국 의료 관광객 유치, 넘어야 할 산 많다. Retrieved from http://www.globalwindow.org/gw/overmarket/GWOMAL020M.html?ARTICLE_ID=2133040&BBS_ID=10.

Lee, K. M. (2009, August 12). 미국 의료보험 한국적용…보험회사들 잇따라 타진. *Koreadaily*. Retrieved from http://www.koreadaily.com/news/read.asp?art_id=891100.

Lee, H. W. (2010, January 6). Medical Tourism is Hallyu too. *Chosun Ilbo*. Retrieved from http://www.chosun.com/site/data/html_dir/2010/01/06/2010010601922.html.

Moon, T. G. (2009, May 22). 한국의 병원으로 환자 모십니다. *The Korea Times*. Retrieved from http://m.koreatimes.com/article/525011.

Oh, Y. H. (2009, October 12). 외국환자 年 20만 유치… '이' 보다 좋은 건 없다. *Chosun Ilbo*. Retrieved from http://www.chosun.com/site/data/html_dir/2009/10/12/2009101200105.html.

Oh, J. Y. (2010, September 1). 중문상고 내년부터 '보건·의료 분야' 특성화고로 전환. *Chosun Ilbo*. Retrieved from http://news.chosun.com/site/data/html_dir/2010/09/30/2010093002309.html.

Park, J. Y. (2009a, April 15). 부산 의료관광 본격 실적 올린다. *Chosun Ilbo*. Retrieved from http://www.chosun.com/site/data/html_dir/2009/04/15/2009041500190.html.

Park, J. Y. (2009b, October 30). 부산·경남: "의료산업 키우자" 상호협력·지원 잇따라. *Chosun Ilbo*. Retrieved from http://www.chosun.com/site/data/html_dir/2009/10/29/2009102901965.html.

Park, H. M. (2011, October 10). 7층서 수술, 17층 체크인 … 부산에 국내 첫 '병원호텔'. *Joongang Ilbo*. Retrieved from http://article.joins.com/news/article/article.asp?total_id=6377531.

Ryu, Jae-In, Chul-Shin Kim, Se-Hwan Jung, and Bo-Mi Shin. (2015). Comparative study on Dental fees of Korea, Japan, Germany and United States. *The Journal of the Korean Dental Association*, *53*(4): 266–274.

Shim, J. W. (2009, December 28). Korea is rising as the hub of plastic surgery. *Joongang Ilbo*. Retrieved from http://news.joins.com/article/3940904.

Shin, S. W. (2014, October 11). 복수국적 45세'로…국적법개정안 발의. *Koreadaily*. Retrieved from http://www.koreadaily.com/news/read.asp?art_id=2882396.

Sohn, J. M. (2012, January 5). 한국 기술 중보다 5년앞서… 역시 성형 한류. *Chosun Ilbo*. Retrieved from http://news.chosun.com/site/data/html_dir/2012/01/04/2012010403258.html?Dep0=twitter&d=2012010403258.

Suh, K. H., Choi, J. Y., Kim, Y. H., Kim, J. S., Jang, J. H., Han, A., & Chae, S. (2012, September 25). 올 추석에만 한국에 2억달러 뿌릴 요우커. *Joongang Ilbo*. Retrieved from http://isplus.live.joins.com/news/article/article.asp?total_id=7105827&ref=mobilehttp://article.joins.com/news/article/article.asp?total_id=9418656&cloc=olink|article|default.

Yoo, S. L. (2010, June 3). 가격은 절반… 한·미 양국서 사용 "보험 에이전트 꼭 참여하세요." *Koreadaily*. Retrieved from http://www.koreadaily.com/news/read.asp?art_id=1040240.

# Index

# About the Author

**Sou Hyun Jang** is a research associate at the Research Center for Korean Community at Queens College. She has completed her Ph.D. in Sociology at the Graduate Center of City University of New York (CUNY). She received her M.A. in Sociology from Columbia University and her B.A. in Sociology from Korea University. As an immigrant scholar, her work has encompassed research on immigrant/minority health, medical transnationalism, and Asian-Americans. Specifically, she is interested in understanding how immigrants as an active entity, not a passive one, utilize their own strategies to cope with health issues in the globalization era. In conducting research in these areas, she has used both quantitative and qualitative methods and has published single-authored articles in *Social Science and Medicine*, *American Journal of Health Behavior*, and *International Journal of Health Services.* Her other articles, which mainly focus on education and religion issues about Asian and Korean Americans, appear in *Sociology of Religion*, *Ethnic and Racial Studies*, and *Sociological Perspectives.*

Lightning Source UK Ltd.
Milton Keynes UK
UKHW01n1358230518
323094UK00001B/23/P

9 781498 563321